Herbal Medicine Guide for Beginners

All you need to know about how to use Medicinal Herbs and Natural Remedies for Self Healing

© Copyright 2018 - All rights reserved.

The information in the following pages is broadly considered to be truthful and accurate account of facts, and as such any inattention, use or misuse of the information in question by the reader will render any resulting actions solely under their purview. There are no scenarios in which the publisher or the original author of this work can be in any fashion deemed liable for any hardship or damages that may befall them after undertaking information described herein.

Additionally, the information in the following pages is intended only for informational purposes and should thus be thought of as universal. As befitting its nature, it is presented without assurance regarding its prolonged validity or interim quality. Trademarks that are mentioned are done without written consent and can in no way be considered an endorsement from the trademark holder.

Table of Contents

Introduction

Congratulations on downloading Herbal Medicine Guide for Beginners and thank you for doing so.

The following chapters will discuss a basic overview of the history of medicinal herbs, from the first man to when herbal medicines became a trading commodity of the world. You will learn the definitions for all of the forms that medicinal herbs can take, what is in the label, and what to look for on the shelf.

There are three chapters providing you with choices of medicinal herbs to treat ailments physically, mentally, and emotionally. Also, we will bring you back to where early man started, being in-charge of your health through the creation of your own medicinal herb garden.

All of the information contained within is practical advice, easy to follow, and designed for your well-being. We encourage you to make medicinal herbs part of your medicine chest and hopefully, part of your everyday health regime. Safer than pharmaceutical options for many of the more common afflictions, medicinal herbs may be the best investment you can make for your future. This guide will lead you into a better quality of life through a deeper appreciation for the world of medicinal herbs.

There are plenty of books on this subject on the market, thanks again for choosing this one! Every effort was made to ensure it is full of as much useful information as possible, please enjoy!

Chapter 1:
A Brief History of Medicinal Plants & Herbs

The English Oxford defines a medicinal plant: *(of a substance or plant) having healing properties.*

Today, a medicinal plant is recognized as one which is used for the maintenance of health and/or to be taken to alleviate a specific ailment. This recognition takes place both in modern and traditional forms of medicine. It was conservatively estimated that there are over 17,810 species of plants which have a use for medicinal purposes out of the 30,000 plants documented for possessing a use of any kind. (The Royal Botanic Gardens, Kew, 2016)

Plants, many of which we recognize today as culinary herbs and spices, have been considered since pre-historic times as containing medicinal value. Humans originated with a close connection to their immediate environment, using what was available to them for food and medicine. Flowering plants are the original source of most medicines. These tended to grow near human settlements, such as chickweed, yarrow, dandelion, and nettles. The trial and error approach was taken when these early 'scientists' applied these sources as potential plants to meet their needs. The knowledge gained was transferred from each generation through oral and written traditions, depending on the culture involved. This knowledge has been gradually becoming more complete as civilizations formed and the sharing of knowledge occurs.

Not only do humans use their environment as a source of medicine, animals including primates, sheep, and monarch butterflies, also consume certain medicinal plants when ill.

The earliest evidence known for the use of plants as medicine comes from prehistoric burial sites. Dating back to the Paleolithic period, a 60,000-year-old Neanderthal site in Iraq contained quantities of pollen from eight plant species, seven of which we use today as remedies.

The earliest written evidence comes from clay tablets dating back to the Sumerian civilization. Recorded on them are hundreds of plants, including opium, used for their medicinal values. Papyrus scrolls from ancient Egypt offer details of eight hundred and fifty plant-based medicines. The source of pharmacopeias, *De materia medica*, documented more than 1,000 medicine recipes based on over six hundred different plant sources. This sourcebook was used for over 1,500 years as a reliable resource for medicinal products.

Before 500 B.C., belief systems at that time ascribed both magical and healing properties to plants. Beginning with the age of Hippocrates, after 500 B.C., physical illness was seen as part of the natural human condition and plants began to lose their mythical properties.

Before the 16th century, there are three widely recognized ancient medicinal systems namely the Chinese medicine, European, and Ayurvedic (Indian). All three are based on very different approaches to the human body but all are in agreement with one essential concept. If the body is out of balance, then illness will result. The restoration of balance is required for good health to be present. One should work with nature and the body's own healing capacity complemented by healing herbs to restore balance.

As part of this shared belief system, all three medical practices held, at their core, a belief that each human contains a primal (vital) energy source. This source sustains the health and life and each individual has it to varying degrees. The Chinese defined this source as "qi" and the Ayurvedic's referred to it as "prana". Westerners referred to it simply as the "vital force".

When world trade exploded in the 14th century, the exchange of remedies and herbs between Muslims, the Chinese, Indians, and Europeans increased. Europeans now add access to new herbs and their healing properties, such as ginger, cinnamon, and cardamom. The Far East was introduced to sage and its potential health benefits at the same time.

Unfortunately, European medicine was not able to treat the many plagues and epidemics that swept through the continent during the 12th and 18th centuries. One common modern day interpretation of the Black plague nursery rhyme *Ring around the Rosie* is that people at the time believed you contracted the disease from breathing 'bad air'. So carrying a posy (sachet) of flowers in your pocket would sweeten the air around you, thus ensuring the carrier would not breathe in any disease.

Herbs brought to Europe from Central and South America, thanks to the Spanish and Portuguese explorers, were potent remedies for successfully treating smallpox, syphilis, and malaria. There followed a surge in popularity for homeopathy and herbal medicines.

In the 19th century, the modern medicine took over, dismissing all previously held concepts of herbal medicine as ignorance and superstition. This was the dawning of the age of western medicine and more traditional practices were overshadowed all over the world.

When the British moved in to colonize India, they declare that the practice of Ayurveda was inferior to western medicine and subsequently tried to squash and replace this traditional form.

China, through the maintenance of closing themselves off the Western world, was more successful at maintaining their traditional medical practices. In many western countries, it became illegal to practice herbal medicine without receiving an official qualification.

People continue to access the healing powers of many plants and herbs, visiting naturopaths, shamans, homeopaths, herbologists, etc. In 1991, the World Health Organization (WHO) formulated a policy on the use of traditional medicines. They have since then published guidelines on the more widely used ones. WHO has estimated, due to a lack of reliable data, up to 80% of our current world population relies on traditional medicine, with approximately two billion of these mainly reliant on medicinal plants. One reason for this is the affordability of plant-based medicines making them more accessible to many people.

In developed countries, there is an increase in the use of plant-sourced medicines which include health care or herbal care products. The benefits from these sources are not always scientifically known as there has been no means of testing the pharmaceutical benefits of each dosage. Since the medicinal value of each plant is dependent on many variables like the soil, sun, a strain of plant, and time of harvesting, it is difficult to assess the benefits and toxicity of these remedies. Although many of these herbal remedies have been in use since early man, there is still very little knowledge of the pharmacological base for their status as a medicinal plant.

Current drug research does make use of ethnobotany to look for active medicinal substances in plants. This research has produced the discovery of hundreds of compounds which are all useful to the medical industry. The most common ones we know of are aspirin (willow bark), quinine, (Remijia bark or Cinchona bark), opium (dried latex from the opium poppy), and digoxin (foxglove flower).

Over a quarter of modern drugs prescribed to patients are sourced from medicinal plants and are rigorously tested prior to use. In some non-industrialized countries, medicinal plants can make up the majority of treatments without the same scientific research. Although there is still little regulation, WHO still does coordinate a network for the safe and practical use of such plants.

Today, there is an annually global export market value of several hundred billion USD in 2017. This market is made up of up to 70,000 plants with anticipated medicinal values. Given that there is little regulation worldwide in the market, medicinal plants face the threat of over-collection to meet demands. Furthermore, climate change and on-going habitat destruction are affecting the viability of these potent medicinal sources. By actively engaging in a deeper awareness of traditional medical knowledge, we can play a key role in a sustained exploitation of these natural resources.

In almost every culture in the world, plants are used as a medical resource. In industrialized nations, the efficacy, safety, and quality of these plants (herbal drugs) have very recently become a key issue. Through the standardization and evaluation of the active plant-derived medical compounds, medicinal plants can assist as an emerging boon to our current healthcare system. Herbal drugs could be the stimulus for future cures of many human diseases. Collaboration with different cultures on their medicinal plant practices is required for the creation of historically accurate accounts for the benefit of the people all over the world.

Beyond their medicinal value, medicinal plants have the potential to increase the quality of life through socio-economic benefits. There is the financial benefit to those who cultivate them for sale, in addition to job opportunities, income via taxation, and a healthier labor force worldwide. The market should be encouraged and further developed through improved practices in the processing and distribution, further scientific research into their medicinal value, and improved financing for those trying to cultivate them.

In the United States most herb product manufacturers already have their products sourced through domestic and foreign markets. The medicinal herb manufacturing industry has been in a steady growth for a number of years and it has matured. Note the number of products readily available in grocery stores, pharmacies, even dollar stores. Probably the best method of purchasing choice organically grown medicinal herb products is by buying products made from from small local manufacturers. Because these companies do not buy in the amounts internationals do they will be the ones purchasing from the local farmer closest to them. By supporting local business you are encouraging diversity and sustainability in the medicinal herb products market.

Chapter 2:
What to Look For In Your Modern Day Medicinal Herbs and Where to Find Them

In this chapter, we will use herb and plant interchangeably with the understanding that an herb is the whole or part of a whole plant which, for the definition of this Guide, is used for its medicinal properties.

Herbal products are defined as being formulated from plants to treat diseases and maintain health. These can come in the form of gels, lotions, salves, ointments, and creams which can be applied directly to your skin. Some products are water soluble and are used in the bath.

There are also essences where the volatile oil of the herb is extracted through a steam distillation. The resulting oil can then be added to your bath, inhaled as a scent, or rubbed on the skin. Some oil like that of oregano is even ingested internally defining this one as a supplement rather than a product.

Poultices and plasters, which involve a soft collection of plant material, are laid on the afflicted body part to relieve the swelling and inflammation. This mass is typically held in place with a cloth.

Herbal supplements are products made from plants and designed only for internal use. These can contain parts of or the whole plant itself. Herbal supplements are sold as pills, tablets, powders, extracts, tinctures, teas, dried, and fresh cuttings of the plant itself.

Pills are used as a general term to define either a capsule or a tablet. They are round and oval, whereas a tablet is flat and circular.

A tablet, which is made up of compressed powder in a solid form, is designed to be cut into two parts.

Capsules contain either a powder or a jelly in a dissolvable gel container. The contents of the capsules are dissolved into the bloodstream immediately.

Teas, also known as infusions, are created by soaking the fresh or dried herbs in hot water and letting them seep. These can then be drunk cold or hot.

A decoction is created by simmering the bark, roots, or berries in hot water for long periods of time. These can also be consumed hot or cold.

Tinctures are created through the soaking of an herb in an alcohol and water solution. This process concentrates and preserves the active ingredients in the herb. Tinctures can vary in their strength and are expressed through a ratio of the weight of the dried herb to the volume of the finished product. Extracts involve soaking the plant in a solvent which removes certain types of chemicals. The resulting liquid can be used as is or evaporated to create a dry powder for use in tablets or capsules.

In 1994, in the United States, the Dietary Supplement Health and Education Act became law. As defined by Congress, a supplement for safe use is one which:

- is used with the intention of supplementing the diet.

- contains one or more of the following as ingredients – herbs, botanicals, amino acids, vitamins, minerals, and other substances,

- the intention is to ingest this orally as a liquid, pill, tablet, capsule, tea, or tincture,

- is clearly and accurately labeled on the front of the bottle as a supplement.

Herbal supplements can range in effect from a mild action with very subtle effects noted over a long period of time to very potent results. Many of the liquid supplements have varying strengths, dependent on if it is a tea, a tincture, or even an extract. A difference in how the supplement is prepared and the concentration of the chemical recovered from the plant can affect the outcome of how it is used. For example, peppermint tea is a fairly mild digestive aid but peppermint oil is very concentrated and can be toxic if not taken correctly. It is important to read the labeling on the supplement or, if you are using the whole herb, consult with a professional for an accurate dosage.

Since the FDA does not consider herbal supplements as drugs (they are classified as food under the Act), they are not subject to the same testing and regulatory standards as drugs. On the labels, the supplements list how the herbs can influence different physical responses but they are not allowed to say they can treat specific conditions.

Determining a manufacturer's claims of quality can depend on hearsay, a doctor's opinion, or even the label itself. Since 2007, there has been something called the Good Manufacturing Process for dietary supplements. These are a list of requirements and expectations which manufacturers have to adhere to for the identification, concentration, purity, and quality of their product. This is in an attempt to prevent the wrongful inclusion of contaminated ingredients, an imbalance of ingredients, and the improper labeling of their product.

We have talked about what to look for when purchasing packaged and prepared medicinal herbs. You can locate these alternatives at health food stores, dietary supplement stores, pharmacies, and even in your big chain grocery stores. While these options are a great alternative to chemicals, there is always the option of creating your own remedies at home. This option will be discussed further in Chapter Six, Growing Your Own Medicinal herbs.

If you do not have the option to garden and want to go pick some herbs, here are a few practical tips to follow.

Rule One. Identify what you are picking correctly. It is extremely easy to confuse some herbs which are indistinguishable in looks but contain very different properties for healing purposes.

Rule Two. Always pick more than a mile off the highway. There are some herbs that seem to thrive on car exhaust fumes. Plants picked next to a busy road may have up to 200 times their natural lead content.

Rule Three. If your herb of choice is growing profusely in a given area, this is a good indication that the soil is nutrient and mineral-rich which is promoting that healthy growth. Picking your herbs from areas such as these is a good choice.

Rule Four. Pick your herbs once the dew has evaporated from the leaves, around mid-morning. Many plants will develop mold after picking if there is any dampness on them.

Rule Five. Select only the best plants, avoiding the ones that display any signs of disease or damage. Drooping leaves, black spots or a discolored stem are all signs that the plant is not a healthy one.

A great advantage to using medicinal herbs as a therapy or health enhancement is that it is totally safe especially when it is administered correctly. Beware of the publicity that erroneously states that medicinal herbs can be swallowed in random amounts without any ill effects occurring. Not only is this incorrect, it is also very dangerous.

Medicinal herbs are safer than current western medications but they still must be taken with the awareness of accurate dosage. Always check with a professional what the correct dosage of medicinal herbs you should be taking. Certain plants used for benign purposes are extremely toxic and can create very harmful side effects if not taken with care. Unless you have the medical certification qualifying you to prescribe medication, do not treat anything more than a minor illness at home. Always talk to professionals about any serious health concerns. If your minor illness is not responding to your medicinal herbal remedies, you should seek professional advice. Keep in mind that if you have any doubts regarding a medicinal herb best not to take it until you can confer with an expert in herbal medicines.

Chapter 3:
External Physical Uses and the Specific Herbs

This chapter will cover six of the more common ailments that can afflict the average human. Although the frequency of these may vary with our age and our physical activity level, most of us will experience at least two of these ailments at least one time in our life.

Cuts and Bruises

Probably the number one cross-generational ailment there is. It is also one of the ones that we can be assured will go away with time.

Arnica is top of the list for its medicinal power. Used for centuries, this pretty plant can be applied topically (cream, essential oil or tincture) for treating bruises and offering some pain relief right at the source. Arnica can also be taken orally as a form of homeopathy, providing healing for physical and emotional trauma.

Comfrey is well respected in permaculture gardens as it reproduces like crazy while improving the soil at the same time. For humans, Comfrey is respected for its active ingredient, allantoin which is a compound that assists with increasing the speed of cellular growth which is extremely beneficial with the healing of cuts, bruises, and even broken bones. Comfrey is normally applied in poultice form.

Chamomile is not only a yummy cup of tea. It is also an anti-inflammatory with antibacterial properties. Wet tea bags can be applied directly to cuts for the best treatment results.

Eucalyptus is known for its consumption by koala bears and the medicinal smell of its leaves. This smell is redolent of the antiseptic properties contained in those leaves making it a good poultice for pain reduction in muscle and joint injuries or used as an ointment for small cuts. If using Eucalyptus in oil form, be sure to dilute it before applying to the affected area.

Plantain can be found all over your yard. You can easily find one if you have been bitten by a bee or spider. Chew a few leaves to get the juices flowing then apply directly to the bitten area, barring that you can find it in a tincture or salve form. Plantain is also useful for bruises and cuts.

Tea Tree oil is known for its antibacterial powers and is used as an antiseptic in hand soaps and antimicrobial in dish soaps. Originating in aboriginal Australia, this oil is very powerful when applied topically as it treats cuts and prevents the risk of infection.

Witch Hazel can be substituted for rubbing alcohol because of its astringent properties causing the damaged tissues to contract and slow or stop bleeding. This will help bruise injuries to fade faster as it speeds up the recovery time of the internal damage. Witch Hazel can be applied by soaking a cotton pad or cloth and applying directly to the area.

Yarrow has been used on battlefields to treat deep puncture wounds. It has both anti-bacterial and anti-inflammatory qualities which work on the wound to both heal and prevent scarring. Yarrow is most often found in tincture or extracts form.

Swelling, Inflammation, & Arthritis

Many of the medicinal herbs available for treating inflamed joints, whether due to injury or arthritis, are taken orally. These treatments will be covered in Chapter 4. The three mentioned here are for external use only. Apply the herb extracts directly to the afflicted area for immediate results.

Aloe Vera is most commonly known for treating small scrapes and minor burns, sunburns or heat burns. The same gel you use on your sunburn can be applied to relieve the ache in your joints.

Frankincense or Boswellia is well-known to herbal medical practitioners for the plant's anti-inflammatory properties. Derived from the Boswellia tree found in India, the gum is believed to work by blocking the substances which attack a healthy joint in autoimmune diseases like Rheumatoid Arthritis. This herb is available in a topical cream form.

Eucalyptus shows up here for the tannins found in its leaves. These tannins are useful in the reduction of swelling and pain in swollen joints. You can follow up an application of Eucalyptus with a heating pad to increase the absorption into the area. This can be found in a topical oil extract. Be sure to dilute it a little with non-medicinal oil before applying directly to the skin.

Capsaicin is the active ingredient in hot peppers. For pain relief, this ingredient works to manipulate physical pain by limiting our perception of pain, triggering endorphins to release, and offering an analgesic action. The lower concentrate creams can significantly reduce arthritic pain while those with a higher capsaicin concentration works well for peripheral nerve pain. Be careful to avoid touching the eyes or other sensitive tissue when using.

Comfrey, added here for a topical treatment for broken bones, is also known as knitbone. Used as a poultice once your bone is out of a cast or if your bone area can be accessed, comfrey leaf can be used dried or fresh, steeped in a little water and oil (to prevent the leaf from sticking to the skin) and applied directly to the skin surface and covered with gauze to hold it in place. For the best results, change the poultice every couple of hours.

Skin Health, Dry & Cracked, Burns, Eczema, Psoriasis, Insect Bites and Acne

The skin is the largest organ in our body. Many of us forget to factor in the regular maintenance of this organ when we think about our overall physical well-being. Some of the following medicinal are specific to certain conditions. Be sure to test for potential allergic reactions by applying a small amount on a part of your body 12 to 24 hours prior to use on the affected area.

Aloe Vera again appears at the top of every medicinal plant practitioners list due to the gel or fluid contained within its leaves being used for centuries as a healing agent and a topical pain-reliever. Aloe can be very effective in treating psoriasis as well as all types of burns and cracked skin.

The Calendula Flower has a history of success in treating rashes and burns and certain kinds of skin ulcers. Calendula tea can be made into a compress as well as using it topically in cream form.

Comfrey roots and leaves have shown themselves useful in the treatment of rashes. Be careful though, a topical application should not last more than three days concurrently as overuse of this plant on the broken skin can lead to toxicity in the area.

The Chamomile flower, both dried and fresh, can be used in tea form as an oral rinse to treat gingivitis and mouth lesions. Externally, chamomile in cream form works to relieve itchy lesions, sunburns, and hives. Chamomile oil mixed with oatmeal in a bath is a soothing skin treatment for eczema.

Lavender, or more specifically, Lavandula angustifolia, is widely recognized for its skin healing compounds. You can find it in cream, ointment, carrier oil, and hydrosol format for almost every skin ailment there is including psoriasis, acne, and irritated skin. You can use it as a facial steam for an anti-aging treatment.

The Marshmallow root is the more common source of this plant to be found in skin and hair formulas. It is both a source of anti-inflammatory and skin-soothing agents helpful for treating eczema, burns and moisturizing dry skin.

Rose water is known for a popular scent most typically ascribed to elderly English females. They might be on to something. Roses contain antibacterial and anti-inflammatory, making them very effective in acne-prone skin. These compounds are richly effective in anti-aging care, nourishing, hydrating, and even rejuvenating skin.

Digestion

Aids for digestion are most commonly taken orally but there is one worth mentioning as an external source of comfort.

Peppermint oil contains menthol, an active ingredient in rubs and liniments. Diluting a few drops into some massage oil (sweet almond) and rubbing over the abdominal area will have a relaxing and anti-spasmodic effect on the smooth muscles of the gastrointestinal tract.

Headaches

Headaches occur for a wide variety of reasons such as tension, dehydration, fatigue, eye strain, allergies, colds, and trauma to name a few. Many of the medicinal plant sourced remedies are taken orally but there are three methods you can try externally to ease the pain. Be sure to drink water as well as trying the following.

Peppermint Oil can stimulate a marked increase of blood flowing to the forehead while soothing muscle contractions. In combination with ethanol, Peppermint Oil can reduce your headache sensitivity. You can dilute this oil with a few drops of sweet almond or coconut oil and rub directly onto your temples, forehead, and the back of your neck.

Lavender Oil is used in this context as a mood stabilizer and very mild sedative. You can place a few drops on a cotton pad or cloth and keep close by, inhaling it every fifteen minutes or so for the best effect. You can also apply the oil in the same method Peppermint oil is used.

Apple Cider Vinegar is not traditionally known as a medicinal plant. However, it is plant sourced and used for the treatment of certain ailments. Pour two cups of the vinegar into a hot bath. This will help draw the uric acid out of your body relieving tension and headaches.

Foot Care

If you are on your feet all day there is nothing like a foot bath to freshen the feet. TI prepare a foot tea, heat one gallon of water to boiling, remove from the heat and add sixteen heaping teaspoons of fresh herb. Cover, allowing to steep for twenty minutes. Strain herbs out and soak your feet. You can also stir five drops of the herb's essential oil into warm water and soak.

Catnip will relax feet that are stressed.

Chamomile, flowers, will relieve swollen feet.

Eucalyptus leaves are deodorizing and energizing.

Ginger Root will warm chronically cold feet.

Horsetail can reduce perspiration.

Juniper is an excellent anti fungal.

Loveage works as a strong deodorizer.

Peppermint can cool feet that feel overheated while energizing tired feet.

Thyme can work as both an antifungal and a foot refresher.

Eye Care

These herbs soothe tired, red eyes while softening the delicate skin around the eye itself. Take care when using herbs around the eyes. Keep the remedy as pure as possible. Below are five herbs you can create a strong decoction with, straining it twice to ensure all little bits are removed from the liquid. Use gauze of flannel to dip in the liquid and squeeze enough so that the cloth is not dripping. Lay down to apply, leaving cloth on closed eyes for fifteen minutes.

Calendula is an extremely gentle herb, very soothing to inner eye and the skin around the outer eye. Use only the flower petals for making the decoction.

Chamomile is very effective to use when your eyes are strained from overuse.

Mallow is a very useful herb. Using as a decoction around the eyes will aid with softening the delicate skin.

Mint can assist with reducing the dark circles

under the eyes. Be careful to not get any into the eye itself when using the decoction. Carefully dab on the skin itself with a cotton ball.

Rose will soothe and calm the skin around the eyes. Be careful to use only organic roses as the ones in floral markets have been sprayed with many chemicals that will harm your skin.

For Cleaning and Refreshing your Home

Lavender is a known disinfectant, mix a little oil with water and it can be applied safely to any surface. This will leave behind a scent which will calm and ease anxiety.

Eucalyptus, Tea Tree and Lavender all possess anti-bacterial properties. You can mix a few drops of all of them in some water to create a general disinfectant which also kills mold.

Lemon juice and Mint mixed together in water will provide you with sparkling windows and a fresh smell that discourages flies from hovering close by.

Chapter 4:
Internal Use

Herbal medicine practices regularly use combinations of herbs designed to work together to increase effectiveness and reduce the side effects of the treatment. The synergy between the active ingredients is a common occurrence in these remedies creating the effect that the therapeutic result is greater than the sum of the ingredients involved. This can be noted in that many medicinal plants show up under multiple categories for healing.

Herbal medicines, when prescribed, are done so with the individual in mind. Dosage, combinations of remedies, and timelines are based on the individual's needs at the time. Be sure to inform yourself of the appropriate dose for your body size and lifestyle.

If you are choosing to treat your minor ailments without medical input, walking into the Natural medicine aisle of your local store can be daunting given the plethora of available options for internal treatments. Having some basic knowledge of what each herb is for can provide you with the tools for choosing the best option for your particular needs. All of the herbs mentioned here can be ingested in powder, capsule, pill, or dried or fresh form. Be careful to always read the recommended dosage on the label or follow the advice given to you by your health practitioner.

Liver and Digestion

Since the times of the Roman Empire, Artichoke has been used as a digestive herb and liver tonic. One of the stronger digestive herbs, it stimulates bile flow, improving digestion, and assisting the body in breaking down food and absorbing alcohol. Artichoke will help alleviate Irritable Bowel Syndrome (IBS), nausea, bloating, and constipation.

Dandelion is used for restoring potassium levels in the body acting as a natural diuretic and promoting a healthy digestive system. Coffee made from roasted Dandelion roots is widely recognized for detoxing the liver while also acting as a tonic. Tea made from dried

Dandelion leaves can assist throughout the day in the body's excretion of excess fluids.

Ginger is an amazing warming spice that is very effective for remedying many of the body's natural functions. Introduced into Europe from China during the times of the Roman Empire, this root has a revered place in traditional Chinese medicine for over 2,000 years. Consumption can alleviate motion sickness, nausea, expel gasses from the gastrointestinal tract, stomach cramps, and heartburn. The root can be purchased and grated into hot water to make a tea. You can incorporate it directly into your food or take it in capsule form for a more powerful effect.

Slippery Elm Bark was used by Native North Americans in poultices while European settlers used it to calm the digestive symptoms of people suffering from typhoid. The inner powdered bark of the elm tree is used today as a common remedy for acid dyspepsia, IBS, or any problem which may occur when you ingest a food that causes discomfort. The moisturizing property protects the stomach lining, easing diarrhea and intestinal cramps while flushing toxic wastes in the intestinal system. It can also be very helpful in healing the stomach lining when leaky gut syndrome occurs.

Milk Thistle, a flowering member of the daisy family, is used for digestion and to strengthen the liver. It has liver-protective powers which mean that it is effective for treating many liver disorders through maintaining the liver cells healthy and neutralizing the effect toxins have on this organ.

Peppermint, noted as an external digestive remedy in Chapter 3, returns here in oral form for relief from colic, a sluggish digestion, bloating, and gas. Peppermint oil is medically accepted as an effective treatment for IBS, as they can assist with easing the symptoms of cramps, bloating and spasms. Ingestion can take the form of infusions or teas and also in capsules for a more direct response to IBS symptoms.

Headaches, Muscle Tension

Butterbur has been effectively used for many years to treat tension headaches. The extract helps to reduce the intensity and frequency of headaches and is effective as a preventative for both adults and children. Butterbur contains both anti-inflammatory and antispasmodic qualities.

Feverfew contains a pain relieving biochemical called parthenopids which are known to limit the dilation of blood vessels on the head, a condition which can be the cause of severe headaches. Feverfew is very effective at minimizing the severity, frequency, and duration of headaches, migrants in particular.

Gingko Biloba is well known as a circulatory stimulant specifically for the brain. It is one of the remedies for ensuring the blood stays fluid due to an anti-platelet activity property which means it is a great source for preventing headaches caused by altitude sickness.

White Willow Bark, the active ingredient in aspirin, is an excellent choice for reducing the pain that comes with tension headaches. It is highly effective and easy on the digestive system and liver making it the preferred choice for over-the-counter choices.

Devil's Claw, from South Africa, is a plant with medicine right in its roots. The plant is very good at relieving muscle tension in the neck, shoulders, and back. It can be taken in tincture or extract form.

Chamomile has 36 flavonoids, compounds which act as an anti-inflammatory. Drinking a cup of Chamomile tea will help reduce the spasms in muscles, thus alleviating pain.

Cherry Juice is very effective at minimizing muscular stress created by physical activity. Tart cherry juice will reduce pain. The antioxidants and anti-inflammatory also assist the muscles to relax to alleviate muscular tension.

Bones & Joints

All joint ailments benefit from an increased intake of essential fatty acids. This can be done by increasing your Omega 3 intake through a variety of oils available or through the supplements listed below.

Burdock Root contains sterols, tannins, and essential fatty acids. These all add up to its reputation as an anti-inflammatory. You can chop up the fresh root and use it in stir fry or make a decoction with the dried root. This herb is also available in capsule form.

Flaxseed Oil is the best option for a vegan source of Omega-3's which are essential to fight inflammation and build a healthy immune system. Note that the body absorbs the oil form much more easily than breaking down the seeds. Never cook flax or heat.

Tumeric is also an extremely effective herb for relieving joint inflammation and an effective pain remedy. It contains at least two of the same compounds found often in prescribed anti-inflammatory. Its effectiveness is the reason why it is readily used for treating cataracts, cancer, and Alzheimer's.

Stinging Nettle is another extremely effective herb used in the treatment of arthritis and gout. Anti-inflammatory properties combined with the minerals boron, calcium, silicon, and magnesium ease pain and assist in the building of a strong bone structure. Taken in leaf tea, it can help to alleviate and decrease water retention and inflammation in addition to fostering the healthy functioning of the kidneys and adrenal glands.

Licorice works very much like the body's own corticosteroids (anti-inflammatories). It can decrease the number of free radicals at the point of injury and inhibit enzyme production, a normal part of the inflammatory reaction. Licorice will also partner with the body's own release of cortisol, a naturally occurring reaction to suppress the immune system, thereby easing pain and arthritic flare-ups. It can also work to inhibit a few of the side effects of cortisol such as adrenal fatigue and resulting anxiety. Licorice can be ingested as a tea or in pill form.

Horsetail is the plant with the highest source of silica, a compound known to improve the integral tissue of the bone. It can assist with bone repair and control calcium absorption. It is best to take this in a three-week on, one-week off cycle to prevent any strain on the kidneys.

Alfalfa leaves are an excellent source of plant-based minerals essential for bone health such as calcium, magnesium, zinc, boron, and silica. The leaf is a good source of phytoestrogens, compounds used to balance out any hormonal fluctuations which can create bone ailments.

Yarrow is used in addition to the two herbs mentioned above as it increases the circulation of blood to the injured area. This is best taken in a tincture or tea form.

Comfrey, otherwise known as knit-bone, is an herb known for its rapid bone healing properties. Taken orally as soon as the injury occurs will assist in a quick recovery.

Red Clover is known to work well for people with osteoporosis due to it being a good source of phytoestrogens and minerals. Research has shown that women taking a regular supplement of red clover isoflavones developed significantly lower rates of spinal bone loss than the subjects in the placebo group.

Heart, Blood and Circulatory System

Cayenne Pepper is a favorite among herbal medical practitioners for increasing blood circulation and as a blood cleanser. As stimulate for the circulatory system, it works by dilating the blood vessels, thus increasing blood flow throughout the body. This herb can be added to your cooking or taken in pill form.

Ginger works as a nice alternative if the cayenne pepper is a bit too strong. This gentle warming herb activates blood circulation by thinning the blood. One Japanese study found it beneficial for improving the blood flow in the intestines themselves. Drinking a few cups of ginger tea each day is a nice way to stimulate your circulation system.

Prickly Ash bark is a very effective remedy for improving poor circulation of the blood resulting in cold hands and feet. The active compounds stimulate the central nervous system improving blood flow throughout the whole body.

Hawthorn has been used for years in the

treatment of heart disease, mild congestive heart failure, and irregular heartbeats. The bioflavonoids occurring in Hawthorn assist in the dilation of blood vessels which protects them from free radicals, generally improving circulation throughout the whole body.

Garlic is one of the most versatile of the medicinal plants. Raw garlic contains high quantities of allicin, used to improve blood flow while also working as a diuretic to flush out excess fluids. Studies out of Britain have shown that garlic tablets increase whole body's blood circulation which results in a reduced risk of heart disease.

Cinnamon is one of the medicinal herbs that has a nice taste and is used to improve the level of blood sugar in the body and circulation. Chinese medicine doctors have accessed Cinnamon for centuries as a warming agent to assist with digestion and circulation.

Coumarin is the active ingredient which contains the compounds for thinning the blood.

Rosemary is known for improving circulation amongst those with muscle pain, sciatica, and neuralgia thereby easing muscle pain. The increased circulatory benefits include skin rejuvenation and are a good supplement for rheumatic ailments.

Yarrow, as mentioned previously, can dilate the capillaries and aids in the toning of the blood vessels themselves. It works by decongesting the capillaries, affecting the flow of blood and stimulating circulation in the body's peripheral areas. When combined with Lime Blossom and Hawthorn, Yarrow works to remedy high blood pressure and prevent blood clots from forming.

Pulmonary Circulatory System

Cinnamon shows up here again as several studies have demonstrated its positive cardiovascular effects. You can take the herb in your food, as a tea, or in pill form.

Eucalyptus's active compound is cineole. The many benefits attributed to this compound are as an expectorant, relief from coughing, soothing sinus passages and fighting congestion. Since Eucalyptus also contains antioxidants, it can also support the immune system during times of illness.

Lungwort is a plant which physically resembles its name and medicinal use. Since the 1600's, Lungwort's compounds have been effectively used to clear congestion, promote lung and respiratory tract health, and guard against organisms which adversely affect respiratory health.

Elecampane, although not well known, has been used by the Greeks, Romans, Chinese, and Ayurvedic practitioners for its soothing effects on the smooth tracheal muscles. The plant's roots contain inulin which soothes the bronchial passageways and pantolactone, an expectorant and anti-cough stimulant.

Lobelia, according to some practitioners, is the single most valuable ingredients in herbal remedies to date. Containing the alkaloid lobeline, Lobelia thins out mucus, thus breaking up congestion. Further, it stimulates the adrenal glands' response to release epinephrine, relaxing the airways, and creating easier breathing. It can also relax the smooth tracheal muscles, an active component in cold and cough remedies.

Osha Root is native to the Rocky Mountains, and North American indigenous cultures have used it for respiratory support for many years. The plant's roots contain camphor, making it one of the essential lung-support herbs. It will increase the circulation to the lungs, making deep breaths occur easily.

Peppermint (oil) can be used to promote free breathing and relax the smooth muscles along the respiratory tract. Peppermint has an antihistamine effect while menthol works very effectively as a decongestant. It is also beneficial for fighting organisms due to it being an antioxidant.

In addition to everything listed above in the Pulmonary Section, here are a few choices for dealing specifically with Hay Fever.

Tinospora Cordifolia is well known in India for relieving allergies, helping to alleviate itching, sneezing, and runny nose.

Timothy Grass (Phelum Pretense) has had many studies done regarding its effectiveness. The studies demonstrate that the pollen extract taken under the tongue can aid in the elimination of hay fever and grass pollen allergy symptoms. When injected, the herb can relieve the symptoms of seasonal allergies. Studies have also supported the belief that if given regularly to children for a few years, it can lower their chances of developing asthma.

Reishi Mushroom or the mushroom of immortality is a powerful herb used for centuries by both Japanese and Chinese medicinal practitioners. Research has shown it to be very effective as an antihistamine, controlling the release of histamines in the body.

Dental Care

For centuries, herbal products have been used in dentistry as antiseptics, antioxidants, antimicrobials, antifungals, antibacterial, antivirals, and analgesics. Medicinal herbs have been very effective in the control of microbial plaque (gingivitis and periodontitis) while aiding in the overall healing processes.

Take one teaspoon each of dried rosemary, peppermint, and lavender. Mix them together well and place in one cup of boiling water. Let steep for fifteen minutes, strain, and cool. It can also be used as a mouthwash for halitosis (bad breath).

Frankincense can be chewed in the form of a gum for promoting good oral health. The compounds contained within the oil-based resin are slowly released into the mouth and digestive tract and is beneficial for their antimicrobial, anti-inflammatory, and anti-tumor qualities. Frankincense in essential oil form is a very effective mouthwash. In powder form, the herb leads to a significant decrease in inflammatory conditions, one being plaque caused gingivitis.

Goldenseal is widely used for gum infection treatment. Most effective as a mouthwash, when combined with Myrrh, can be a powerful antimicrobial to be used in cases of acute gingivitis.

Echinacea Root is an American Native remedy for a toothache. The root contains high levels of inflammatory.

Lamiaceae Herbs which include rosemary, mints, lavender and sage are all powerful tools for oral and dental health. They can be used in essential oil form (very aromatic) in mouthwashes and dry powder form for brushing. The leaves of the Sage plant are excellent when used fresh and applied to suppress bleeding of the gums, gingivitis, and sores in the mouth. Peppermint leaves can be chewed fresh for improvement of the breath and to alleviate inflammation of the gums.

Prickly Ash bark is a proven method to stop toothaches or any other mouth pain. It can quicken healing after a pulled or accessed tooth as it improves circulation to the mouth.

Women's health

Women have relied on medicinal herbs for thousands of years, long been known as the practitioners of herbal medicine. The accumulated knowledge from their passing on of this knowledge has brought the practice of herbal medicine to where it is today. Herbs play a significant role in providing support to a woman as she transitions through the periods of her life.

Dandelion is one herb that humans will never be without. It is a powerful tool as a diuretic for pre-menstrual bloating and combined with Stinging Nettle, works together to purify the blood. Dandelion root can be taken in the usual variety of pill forms or taken in coffee form.

Chaste Tree Berry is one of the best for providing support to a woman during her menstrual cycle. It acts as a hormone balancer through the support of the communication between the ovaries and the brain resulting in a healthy level of estrogen and progesterone in the body. This herb should be taken in tincture form.

Red Clover has the densest source of phytoestrogens which are useful when the body's natural estrogen levels are low, for example during menopause. This is useful for other menopausal symptoms such as hot flashes, night sweats, and vaginal dryness due to drops in estrogen levels. The fresh herb can be steeped in a tea and consumed as needed.

Black Cohosh flower essence is the most commonly prescribed herb for menopause. It can be combined with Red Clover to manage symptoms in addition to lifting one's mood. This root can be taken as a tincture, tea, or in capsule form.

Holy Basil (Tulsi) assists with lowering stress hormones (cortisol). It is very calming and can help with mental clarity. This is perfect for mothers who multi-task and are under a lot of stress. Holy Basil is a delicious tea and is used in tincture and capsule form as well.

There are some medicinal herbs which should never be taken with prescription medicine. The potentially fatal health effects are not something to ignore. This warning is given repeatedly and really should be actively followed. The is not to say that if you are taking prescription medication you can not ingest any medicinal herb supplements. Rather be mindful and always research the combinations before administering.

Some potentially adverse combinations include:

St. John's Wort and antidepressants – it can raise the serotonin levels in your body too much potentially leading to seizures, pregnancies in women on oral birth control and inhibited effectiveness of anti-cancer medication.

Fenugreek, can lower the blood sugar level too much and interfere with some medications for diabetes. Also it is a dangerous combination with anticoagulants (warfarin) because Fenugreek can also delay blood clotting.

Gingko Biloba, if taken with aspirin, fish oil or ibuprofen – all blood thinners, can increase the risk of bleeding. Gingko Biloba slows the clotting action of blood and can cause bleeding to occur.

Echinacea will counter act with prednisone. The steroid decreases the immune system while Echinacea stimulates it. You will receive no benefit from either if taken at the same time.

Chapter 5:
Emotional Health

Medicinal herbs are often thought of as treatments for what physically ails us, boost our immune system, alleviate pain, fix our digestive problems and overall, support our physical wellbeing. It is well known that our physical body and our mental/emotional bodies are intertwined. What is happening in one will affect the other two. Both Chinese and Ayurvedic medicine practices support the theory that you cannot address an ailment without looking at all three areas of your life.

When using medicinal herbs to improve your emotional well being, look for ones that include hormone balancing properties and improve liver and gallbladder function. It is always best to work with an experienced herbal practitioner when taking herbs for mentally therapeutic purposes with deep roots. The following have been selected for their use to relieve anxiety, lift your mood, promote sleep and calmness, and to improve focus or clarify mental functions.

Sleep Aids

Lemon Balm, when consumed in tea form, has been traditionally used to treat insomnia and anxiety. It is more recently found to calm people with Alzheimer's disease who suffer from agitation.

Valerian is frequently combined with Lemon Balm, creating a mild but effective sedative for people who struggle with insomnia. It can also be taken on its own in tea form.

Catnip appears to have the opposite effect on humans that it has on cats, as humans only experience calming effects. These include relief from stress and anxiety, helps with migraines, and assists in the treatment of insomnia. You can mix the catnip with chamomile leaves to strengthen its relaxing power.

Anxiety and Stress

The herbs mentioned above are effective for responding to and improving anxiety and stress. Their only drawback is they are also effective sleep aids. The following listed here are also effective without creating drowsiness.

Lavender is a very popular herb used to calm the nerves. Essential oils can be used in a diffuser, scenting your surroundings in tranquility or placing the herb in a sachet to place under your pillow. Lavender scented creams can be applied and there are some who believe ingesting Lavender in pill form will help to reduce anxiety.

Passionflower, taken as a tea, can improve symptoms of anxiety, aviation, and irritability. It is also useful when experiencing opiate drug withdrawal symptoms.

Ashwagandha showed similar effects as those of the pharmaceutical drug lorazepam. A 2012 study showed that taking the plant extract in capsule form can significantly reduce cortisol levels without any serious side effects occurring.

Depression

St. John's Wort is the most prevalent herb used for the treatment of both anxiety and depression. It is well established as an effective anti-depressant, equivalent to those pharmaceutically created, with fewer side-effects.

Maca has been used in Peru for centuries to alleviate depression in men and women while increasing their libido. Some current research has found it very effective for treating symptoms of depression in women going through menopause. The plant is grouped according to its color, but the roots from all of the plants (black, red, cream) are helpful in treating this condition. Maca can be taken in tea or capsule form.

Ginseng has been a staple in the Chinese medicine chest for centuries. The modern-day root is derived from the American or the Asian plant. The qualities it possesses for reducing depression are that it boosts energy and improves mental clarity while reducing the symptoms of stress. These can help people suffering from reduced energy and motivation due to depression. Take note, people with bipolar disorder can trigger mania if taking ginseng.

Chamomile was studied in 2012 for its role in managing depression. The results showed that this herb does produce relief from symptoms of depression, perhaps through its action as a sleep aid. People have more energy and feel fewer symptoms.

Memory and Mental Clarity

Sage has long been known to sharpen the mind. There have been a number of recent studies to support this claim. Common as a Mediterranean culinary herb, Sage can improve mood and memory with a single dose and possibly protect memory and cognition functions in the brain.

Rosemary, another culinary herb from the Mediterranean, can improve cognitive function in low doses. Studies of the herb in aromatherapy use showed that the scent can aid memory and increase focus while reducing stress. Like Sage, Rosemary can also pick up your mood and protect your brain.

Gingko, taken in leaf extract form, is popular in Europe for treating a wide variety of conditions including memory loss and problems associated with concentration and confusion. Gingko is believed to work through the actions of increasing the blood supply, a reduction in blood viscosity and free radicals, and an increase in the presence of neurotransmitters.

Chapter 6:
Growing Your Own Medicinal Herbs

Gardening and herbal medicine are both age-old practice's that have been with us for thousands of years. It is interesting to note that growing the medicinal herbs produces the same benefits as taking them. Gardening can reduce stress, bolster the immune system through exercise and fresh air, keeps your mind sharp, and helps you sleep at night. The benefits of growing your own medicinal herbs are limitless, it's no wonder so many people are turning to grow their own.

The science of gardening continues to develop and with it, the art of healing with herbs. Both have gained popularity due to concerns over our current food sources and the affordability in creating one's own food and medicine source. The availability of information on plant culture, do-it-at-home recipes for herbal remedies, and new research on the multiple uses of these remedies are creating huge potential for growth for all concerned.

In the past, it was common to devote a section of the yard for growing flowers, fruit, vegetables and herbs. These plots were an integral part of the community landscape, socializing with the neighbors over the garden fence was an integral part of a family's everyday life. Frequently, sections of these gardens were wholly devoted to the growth of plants for the purpose of home remedies.

In addition to gardens being a source of the community social fabric, they also created a link between people and nature. Habitats were created to nurture the presence of insects, butterflies, birds and snakes, all necessary for plant pollination and garden health. People kept a closer watch on the weather, relying on their joints to tell them what was going to happen. By digging up a small plot in our yard, or planting pots to set on the balcony, a medicinal herb garden is an active means of staying involved with the natural world around us.

The best advice to be given is, if you are starting an herb garden for your very first time, it is always a wise choice to keep things simple. Start small, maybe five to ten plants. Make it manageable, keep it enjoyable. That way, you will enjoy gardening, finding it pleasurable and not a chore. Plants pick up on their surroundings and beautiful, healthy gardens are built by people who love being in them.

Before you start digging and planting, there are a few considerations to make. Obviously, if you are growing the plants in pots on a balcony, you will have fewer options in respect to sunlight and water source. One of the biggest mistakes you can make is to build your garden far away from a water source. It might seem appealing and back-to-the-earth appealing in the beginning, but hauling water, compost, and tools become very tiring over a season. Try to consider the distance from water to beds (or pots), access for a wheelbarrow to move compost in and weeds out, distance to the compost pile (if you are creating your own) and distance from your house. Of course, much of this will be pre-determined by your lot size but it is good to think of these points and create the most accessible herb plot you can.

The last considerations are sun and soil. How much sun will the plants receive in one day? Most medicinal herbs (not all, but most) would prefer to enjoy up to eight hours of sunshine a day, if not more. More sunshine will result in a higher concentration of oil inside the herb, creating a more potent plant. In respect to soil, is it acidic and filled with rocks? Clay? Sand? Some herbs prefer the Mediterranean conditions of a dry, less loamy soil with excellent drainage while other plants need a cool, shady environment. You can always amend the soil prior to planting, adding compost, peat moss, lime, and bone meal. Be sure to know once you have selected which plants you want to begin your garden with and research the soil and sun requirements prior to planting. This holds true if you are using containers.

One way to strategize the most effective garden is to draw it out. Whether it is round, oval or shaped like a kidney, pick something you will enjoy looking at. Select which medicinal herbs you would like to grow, look at their sun and soil requirements, and then research their growth patterns. Tall herbs will go in the back or the center of the bed or pot. Smaller herbs are placed at the front. If the plant likes to spread, make sure you leave enough room around for adequate growth. This map will help you remember what you have planted from year to year (some herbs are cut right back at the end of the growing season) and it is easy, as the garden grows, to forget what you have planted where.

One way to determine how healthy your soil is by looking for signs of earthworms. If it is a cool day and there are no worms just below the soil surface, you will need to add compost and a little sand to create better drainage for the plants. Organic compost will create healthy plants. Well-aged manure is very effective if it is at least a year old. Note that herbs will develop root rot easily as most of them prefer drier conditions so beware to not overwater in your zeal to get the plants growing.

Next, decide if you are going to start from seeds or buy seedlings. Seeds are less expensive to purchase. You can sprout them inside the house. Add a little organic soil to the cups inside an egg carton, a label of which seeds you have planted where, and place the carton on an old cookie sheet as the water will seep through the cardboard. Place these in a sunny and warm area of the house and in about three weeks, you will have sprouts. By planting more than you need, you will have choices of which plant looks the healthiest.

If you choose to buy seedlings to plant right away, make sure to pick the healthiest looking plants. Garden seedlings are often ready to plant the week you purchase them, so be careful to not leave them sitting in their pots for too long. Ask before you leave the store if the seedlings have been 'hardened off". This phrase refers to if the plants have been outside yet. Typically, planting occurs at a time of year where the air and ground are warmer, but it is best to acclimatize your plants to the outside by leaving them outside for a few hours a day until they are used to the temperatures. You will need to do this with the seedlings you have sprouted yourself.

Plant your seedlings at least two inches apart, more if they will grow into large sprawling plants. Mint should always be planted in a large pot as it will take over your yard in a couple of years. Oregano also has a tendency to spread out and take over. It could also be easily contained in a pot. Fill the hole with a little water, gently place the seedling in the hole, and gently press the dirt done around it. Add a little more water and take a photo – your first medicinal herb garden. It will never look this sparse again.

You can choose to plant the seeds directly into the soil. If so, make sure all risk of frost is past and the soil is reasonably warm. Keep an eye out for birds and rodents, they like to watch what you are doing then follow behind and snack on the seeds.

Medicinal plants which grow very well in pots are basil, calendula, cayenne peppers, ginger, lavender, lemon balm, mint (all varieties), rosemary, sage, St. John's wort and thyme. Note that rosemary does not enjoy being transplanted. They can grow quite large so ensure that the space designated for them is large and they can live there forever. All of the others can be transplanted easily.

Some people plant herbs in concrete building blocks, this keeps the plant's roots warm and keeps them separate, also cuts down on the weeding. Another idea is to lay an old wooden ladder down on a bed and plant a different plant between each rung.

You can plant all of the above container plants in a bed along with chamomile, garlic, feverfew, echinacea, and licorice.

Chickweed, dandelion, and plantain will show up in your yard without too much effort on your part. If you are an apartment dweller, simply visit a field far away from any roads or factories, and you will locate a large assortment of these medicinal plants growing wild.

Plants requiring a fair bit more space to grow as they get big are yarrow, valerian, mullein, burdock, and marshmallow.

Most of the medicinal plants mentioned will have the desire to spread out and take over. At the end of the growing season, ensure there is adequate space around each plant for room to grow the next season. It is very important to be a bit ruthless as healthy plants are the ones with adequate access to water and sunshine. If they are competing with others in the garden, you may lose one or two quieter herbs to more dominant varieties.

Your herbs might be in a competition for garden space but you should never feel you are competing for a gardening award. Keep in mind that if you are not enjoying gardening, you will not be reaping the peripheral benefits of having a medicinal herb garden. Harvesting your own herbs for use in your home should be a gratifying experience, allowing you to continue developing your garden and the options of remedies it can provide you with.

At varying times through the summer, you will be harvesting flowers, leaves. or roots from your plants for the creation of your home remedies. What follows is a basic guide to follow for the proper harvesting techniques to ensure you have the best quality materials from which to create your recipes.

You will only need to harvest the whole plant if you are requiring the roots. Otherwise, you should always only take only small amounts from each plant until your garden is well established. Then, larger harvests can be successfully undertaken as your plants will be hardy enough to sustain a larger leaf/flower loss without destroying the plant. Newer plants will only handle smaller harvesting as they are too small to sustain a whole-scale loss of leaves or flowers.

Flowerheads are prone to damage, from insects, birds, wind, or absentminded gardeners. Try to pick flowers in the morning and dry them at the first opportunity to prevent mold from growing. Any blooms that are already starting to lose their petals are past their prime and should be avoided.

Choice leaves for picking are the ones which have a healthy appearance. Biannual plant leaves should only be selected in their second year.

When you have harvested the parts of the plant you need, leaves, flowers, and seeds, store them in small cotton bags with wire frame placed inside so the leaves are not crushed or damaged.

Never mix two herbs in the same bag. They can look entirely different in your kitchen than they can in the field.

You will now need to prepare your herbs for storage as soon as possible. This is to prevent mold and mildew from growing, whereby you will have to throw out the herbs. There are many ways to preserve medicinal plants and master herbalists will each have their own method. The simplest way to store herbs is to dry them. By removing moisture from the plant, you will trap the active compounds or useful chemicals inside the plant body. This makes the plant immune to disease, mold, and other problems. Dried herbs may be stored for anywhere from three to five years without losing any of their inherent value as medicinal plants.

There are two methods for drying herbs, inside an oven or outside in the sun on a frame. The inside method is quicker, approximately one hour inside the oven as opposed to six weeks outside on the frame.

With oven drying, you will need to place your herbs on a clean, dry tray. Place a piece of aluminum foil, shiny side down, over the tray. Tuck the foil around the tray leaving only a small gap to allow moisture to escape.

Heat the oven to 150 degrees and place the tray in the oven. Take the tray out every fifteen minutes to turn the herbs over so the moisture is being evenly drawn out of the plant. When moisture is drawn out of the plant unevenly, then burning will occur. Do not let this happen. Should the plants turn brown or black, then all potency is destroyed and the plant will be useless to you.

It is very easy to over-dry or burn the plants. If you can crumble the finished, dried plant easily in your hand without it becoming powder and most, if not all, of the original color is intact, the plant is dried perfectly.

A disadvantage to this method is that herbs will lose between one-third and-one half of their potency. When the plants are dried on a frame outside, they only lose one-quarter of their original medicinal value.

For this reason, frame drying is the preferred method by experienced herbalists though it is far more time-consuming. For this option, you will require a small wood or metal box, about three-feet square, with a glass line. Line the base of the box with aluminum foil and leave a small sheltered hole for moisture to escape. Pat dry the selected herbs for drying and place on the foil, closing the lid afterward. The herbs will require turning once a day until dry, anywhere between three to six weeks.

The box should be placed in a spot with adequate sunlight and be watertight. One herb placed in the box still slightly damp will ruin the whole batch.

How you will store your herbs is determined by the method you will be using them. Ointments require powdered forms of the plant while tinctures and teas require whole roots, leave or flowers. So, a good guide to follow is that your leaves and stems are best ground, then stored while the flowers, roots, and seeds are stored whole. Be sure everything is dried thoroughly before storage.

Grinding your herbs into a powder can be done with a mortar and pestle, slower but it does allow you to decide the quality of the powder with a great deal of accuracy. An electric grinder (such as a coffee grinder) gives better uniformity to the finished product and a very fine powder.

You have now arrived at the most important step in the process. Failing to store your herbs correctly will mean you will not be able to use them. This means that all of your time and effort has been wasted.

Choose your storage room carefully. Preferably not damp, cold, or drafty nor near the kitchen as odors from cooking have been known to seep through the most airtight of containers. Never store your herbs within reach of children, they are medicine.

Choose a glass (preferably colored to keep light out), ceramic or earthenware container that is intact and airtight. Do not use anything that will allow sunlight or moisture to seep in.

Take the time to label the container carefully, as failure doing so can have fatal consequences. You should always detail the following information on the labels:

- The date when you picked the herbs. This allows you to track its potency and renew your stocks as required.

- The name of the herb, including the Latin and the common name.

- The method of drying. Since potency is affected by this, it is essential that you know the method to determine the quantity for your remedies and dosage.

- The part of the herb you have stored in the container. Ground up herbs can pretty much all look the same, though the medicinal qualities of the plant vary with the part it is contained. It is very important to know which part you have stored for use.

You are now ready to begin applying your own medicinal herbs for health and symptom relief.

Conclusion

Thank you for making it through to the end of Herbal Medicine Guide for Beginners. Let's hope it was informative and able to provide you with all of the tools you need to achieve your goals whatever they may be.

The next step is to go out and identify some of the more common medicinal herbs growing wild around you. Check out the produce department and notice the variety of the herbs available, fresh and dried. Scan your supplement aisles and acquaint yourself with the varieties of remedies available, the variation in doses, and the range of ailments which can be treated.

Next, walk around your house. Do you have space for a small plot or a few containers? Start researching how much sun your plot would get in a day and what kind of soil you have. Take stock of your medicine cabinet and notice the contents. What do you seem to require the most of in your household? Maybe plan on planting a few herbs that would meet the most common of your household requirements, cuts, bruises, insomnia.

Take your paper and start building your medicinal herb bed map so that when the next growing season arrives, you are prepared to plant your very own ingredients for those herbal remedies.

Finally, if you found this book useful in any way, a review on Amazon is always appreciated!

This book belongs to a series of books about herbal medicine and how to use it to improve our life. For more information, visit www.db-publishing.com

Physical Pain Herbal Medicine

The 10 Best Solutions to Relieve Back, Neck, and Shoulder Pain

© Copyright 2018 by - All rights reserved.

The follow eBook is reproduced below with the goal of providing information that is as accurate and reliable as possible. Regardless, purchasing this eBook can be seen as consent to the fact that both the publisher and the author of this book are in no way experts on the topics discussed within and that any recommend-dations or suggestions that are made herein are for entertainment purposes only. Professionals should be consulted as needed prior to undertaking any of the action endorsed herein.

This declaration is deemed fair and valid by both the American Bar Association and the Committee of Publishers Association and is legally binding throughout the United States.

Furthermore, the transmission, duplication or reproduction of any of the following work including specific information will be considered an illegal act irrespective of if it is done electronically or in print. This extends to creating a secondary or tertiary copy of the work or a recorded copy and is only allowed with an expressed written consent from the Publisher.

All additional rights reserved.

The information in the following pages is broadly considered to be a truthful and accurate account of facts, and as such any inattention, use or misuse of the information in question by the reader will render any resulting actions solely under their purview. There are no scenarios in which the publisher or the original author of this work can be in any fashion deemed liable for any hardship or damages that may befall them after undertaking information described herein.

Additionally, the information in the following pages is intended only for informational purposes and should thus be thought of as universal. As befitting its nature, it is presented without assurance regarding its prolonged validity or interim quality. Trademarks that are mentioned are done without written consent and can in no way be considered an endorsement from the trademark holder.

Table of Contents

Introduction

Congratulations on downloading *Physical Pain Herbal Medicine* and thank you for doing so.

Herbal medicine, which is sometimes called herbalism or botanical medicine, involves using plants, or parts of them, to treat illnesses or injuries. This also includes using botanicals or herbs to help a person's overall health and wellness. Traditional medicine practitioners, herbal medicine practitioners, herbalists, and naturopathic, homeopathic, and Ayurvedic healers all use herbal remedies.

Ginkgo biloba is one of the oldest herbs in history. According to fossil records, Ginkgo has been on the earth since, at least, the Paleozoic period. One of the earliest known medical documents was recorded by the Egyptians around 1500 BC, known as *Papyrus Ebers*. This 20-meter long scroll held 700 plant-based remedies.

Shennong Bencaojing, the first recorded herbal study, was written by the Chinese Emperor Shen Nong around 2000 BC. He was known for his multitude of innovations like dietary revolution, seed preservation, and he had tasted hundreds of herbs. His writings contain information and descriptions for 300 plants.

The monks, during the Middle Ages, grew medicinal herbs. The Native Americans gave the colonist herbs and plants like Black Cohosh, which is still used to relieve pain and menopause symptoms 'till this day.

The extracts, flowers, roots, bark, stems, leaves, and seeds of plants have been used in herbal medicine for more than a millennia. These types of treatments have been given in capsules and pills, in liquid forms, as topical applications, in tinctures and teas, and raw. At first, the plants were all consumed raw or mixed with hot water as a tea or soup. In later years, people started drying and crushing the plants for other uses. The plants were discovered in the wild, and they often based their uses on superstitious or visual cues. People would often use plants to treat body ailments because it looked like that body part or because they commonly grew in a certain area. Science helped people to refine the use of herbal remedies. Herbs and various plants are the precursors to a number of modern medicines.

Today there are many modern and Western medical practitioners that turn to herbal remedies for common and uncommon disorders. The lower cost and safer use are very attractive to medical professionals. There are also some physicians who use herbs to help offset the side effects of regular pharmaceuticals.

There isn't an exact date as to when humans started to use herbs for medicinal purposes. We do know that the first written information about herbal medicine dates back to around 2800 BC in China. Since then, the popularity of herbs for pain relief has gained and fallen out of favor several times in the medical field. The following timeline will show you some of the major points in the history of herbal medicine:

- 2800 BC – The first written information regarding herbal medicine.

- 400 BC – The Greeks started to use herbal medicine. Hippocrates stressed out how important overall happiness, exercise, and diet are as the foundation of wellness.

- 50 AD – The Roman Empire started to share herbal medicine throughout the Empire, and with this started the commerce of cultivating herbs.

- 200 AD – The first appearance of a classification system that paired common illnesses with their remedy. This was created by Galen, an herbal practitioner.

- 800 AD – Monks became the rulers of the herbal field with their gardens in infirmaries and monasteries that cured the injured and sick.

- 1100 AD – The new center of medicinal influence was the Arab world. Physician Avicenna wrote the *Canon of Medicine*, which mentioned herbal medicine.

- 1200 AD – The Black Death started the spread throughout Europe, and herbal medicines were used along with the "modern" methods like mercury, arsenic, purging, and bleeding with similar or better, results.

- 1500 AD – Parliament and Henry VII promoted and supported herbalists and herbal medicine, mainly because of the number of untrained apothecaries that gave substandard care.

- 1600 AD – The poor were treated with herbs, while extracts of animals, plants, mineral, and the "drugs" were given to the rich.

- 1700 AD – Preacher Charles Wesley gave herbal medicine another high-profile endorsement. He was an advocate of herbal treatments, sensible eating, and good hygiene for healthy living.

- 1800 AD – Herbal treatments took a back seat from pharmaceuticals. As the drugs side effects started to be documented, herbal remedies gained popularity. The National Association of Medical Herbalists was created, and then later changed its name to the National Institute of Medical Herbalists.

- 1900 AD – During WWI there was a lack of drugs available, and this increased the use of herbal medicines. When the war ended, penicillin was discovered, and pharmaceutical production increased. Practitioners of herbal medicine had their rights to dispense medication taken away and then reinstated. People started to become concerned about the dangerous side effects and environmental impact of pharmaceutical drugs during the '50s.

- 2000 AD – The EU started to regulate and test herbal medicines, like the regulations in pharmaceuticals.

For nearly 4000 years herbal medicines have been documented. This type of medicine has survived real world testing and thousands of years of human use. There are some medicines that are not used anymore because of their toxicity, while others have been combined or modified with additional herbs to help offset side effects. Herbs have undergone changes in terms of how they are used.

Herbal medicine is still popular today. In some ways, it has even gained new momentum. More and more people have started to seek out alternative treatments. As physicians look for new treatments for the most common illnesses, they are starting to look back at herbal medicines.

Typically, today, herbs are cultivated for medicinal purposes. Very few herbs are harvested in the wild, except for those that are located in higher elevations or rainforests.

Elderly people tend to metabolize medications differently and typically take more medications. This means that they need to exercise caution when they try new herbal supplements.

Pain Relief

There isn't a single herb, vitamin, or mineral that offers the same significant level of pain relief that heavy-duty prescription drugs provide. But, natural herbs for pain relief don't come with the side effects of prescription drugs. They are also more cost-effective and don't come with the same risk of chemical dependency.

Certain herbs not only alleviate pain but also address the underlying causes of it and supports and heals the nervous system. There are over 100 herbs for pain relief, and not all of them work the same. Herbal remedies are meant to work alongside with regular pain treatment.

Over 40% of Americans, according to Johns Hopkins University, use alternative medicinal therapies to help control pain when prescription medications aren't working.

Herbal treatments provide individuals who don't have access to pain clinics access to pain relief. According to researchers from the University of Michigan Health System, the most frequent users of alternative pain management are older individuals.

Herbal remedies tend to be less expensive than conventional treatments. There are also a few side effects, although that doesn't mean there aren't any reactions. Depending on the condition or medication that a person is undergoing, they can have a reaction to herbal remedies. This is why it is important to speak to your health care provider first and do plenty of research.

Before we dive into the book, a word of advice, make sure that you talk to your doctor before you start trying any of these alternative pain relief methods. While they are all natural, there is a chance you could be allergic to them, or they could interact with any prescriptions you are taking. I have tried to add in as much information on possible problems, but there could be more than I am unaware of.

There are plenty of books on this subject on the market, thanks again for choosing this one! Every effort was made to ensure it is full of as much useful information as possible, please enjoy!

Capsaicin

A big part of the cuisine in India, Central America, and Asia are chili peppers. In the United States, you can go to any store that sells sauces and find a variety of hot sauces oftentimes with the words "fire," "inferno," or "insanity" on the label.

People love chili peppers because of this heat, and it's also the biggest reason why it has so many medicinal properties, particularly pain relief. The capsaicin found in chili pepper is what gives it its heat. Capsaicin is a compound that the chili pepper produces to protect the pepper from fungal attack. Capsaicin is odorless and colorless, but when consumed, it makes your brain believe that there is heat wherever it comes in contact with your body.

Interestingly, though, birds aren't affected by capsaicin. This makes it possible for them to spread the seeds around so that the plant can survive. Virtually all mammals are affected by capsaicin, although, it's believed that humans are the only mammals who willingly choose to eat them.

How Peppers Tricks the Brain

The nervous system has TRPV1 receptors, which are heat-receptor proteins. These are located in the cells of your digestive system and skin. The receptors are inactive unless a person is exposed to temperatures over 107.6 degrees Fahrenheit.

Once this happens, you will experience pain and heat, which is telling you that you need to move away from whatever is causing this heat. When a person eats a chili pepper, the capsaicin in it will bind to and activate TRPV1. This means that though there isn't any real danger, your body believes that it's being exposed to excessive amounts of heat.

The *New York Times* further explains this:

"... in mammals it stimulates the very same pain receptors that respond to actual heat. Chili pungency is not technically a taste; it is the sensation of burning, mediated by the same mechanism that would let you know that someone had set your tongue on fire."

The Scoville scale is used to measure the intensity of heat in peppers; it was developed by Wilbur Lincoln

Scoville in 1912. Bell pepper is ranked as zero on the Scoville scale; pure capsaicin is ranked at over 15 million SHU.

A jalapeno pepper ranges from 2500 to 8000 SHU, and a Scotch Bonnet pepper measures as high as 350,000. Ghost chilies, one of the hottest peppers, measure around 900,000 SHU.

Burning Sensation Equals Pain Relief

Capsaicin is able to help alleviate pain mainly by getting rid of what is known as substance P. This is a chemical component of all of the nerve cells that work to help transmit pain signals to the brain. The same substance is also what de-sensitizes the sensory receptors in the skin.

This is the reason why it is commonly added to cream that is used as a topical pain relieving medicine, as well as in patches, which can sometimes be ranked as 10 million SHU. Ironically, the very intense burning sensation is what provides the pain relief.

Capsaicin is most often used for relieving pain associated with shingles and HIV neuropathy, but it is also very helpful in relieving all types of joint pain including neck, back, and shoulder.

One research study examined a man who had persistent pain because of the wounds he received from a bomb explosion, and he was able to experience an 80 percent reduction in pain after using an 8% capsaicin patch.

A low concentration, 0.025%, topical capsaicin cream is helpful in relieving the pain caused by osteoarthritis. 80% of patients were able to experience a reduction in pain after only two weeks of four-times a day treatment.

It has also been found to help in reducing or eliminating the redness, itching, stinging and burning of skin due to moderate to severe psoriasis. A 2009 study examining a nasal spray that contained capsaicin found that it was able to significantly reduce allergy symptoms.

How is Capsaicin Used?

There are two main forms of capsaicin:

Capsaicin cream – This is common for most types of pain relief. Doctors will often suggest creams, ointments, films, sticks, gels, ointments, or lotions. These do not require prescriptions. This form will be thoroughly rubbed into your skin in the area where you are hurting and reapplied throughout the day. Make sure that you thoroughly wash your hands after you use the cream. Make sure the cream doesn't go near your mouth or eyes, or any other mucous membrane.

Capsaicin patches – This has higher amounts of capsaicin than the cream. This is often suggested by doctors for shingles pain and diabetic neuropathy. These can only be acquired from doctors. The doctor will numb the area and then apply the patch. This normally takes around two hours.

This patch has the ability to help relieve pain for up to three months. Avoid messing with the patch while it is on.

Side Effects

While capsaicin is fairly safe, the patches and creams can irritate the skin and cause some of the following:

- Pain

- Itching and burning

- Dryness

- Soreness

- Swelling and redness

This will often become worse in humid and hot weather, when bathing in warm water, and when sweating, but typically only lasts for a couple of days but can last for two to four weeks.

You will need to make sure you use sunscreen because capsaicin can make your skin more sensitive to heat and sun. Some people can be allergic to capsaicin. Contact your doctor if you experience trouble breathing, chest tightness, swelling in your throat, hives, and itching.

There are rare side effects from using the patch that can affect your heart, but these include a sudden increase or decrease in heart rate and blood pressure changes. Make sure your doctor knows your history of any heart problems, blood vessel problems, or if you suffer from high blood pressure.

Turmeric

Chances are you, have probably heard people rave over the health benefits of turmeric. There are loads of research that looked further into the vitamins and macronutrients in foods to phytochemicals and micronutrients.

The majority of the benefits of turmeric come from its anti-inflammatory and antioxidant potential and its ability to create homeostasis in the body. Because of this, people have started to turn towards eating healthful whole foods again, and turmeric's curcumin is the heaviest hitter when it comes to phytonutrients.

For example, curcumin has been found to be more effective than celecoxib to treat arthritis pain. Curcumin has antifungal, antioxidant, and antiviral properties. It also works to inhibit the function of molecules that cause inflammation because it contains COX-2 inhibitors. COX-2 is an enzyme that causes the formation of prostanoids, which is a fatty acid that causes an inflammatory reaction. This is also influenced by chronic inflammation caused by metabolic oxidation that the body goes through every day, local inflammation caused by minor injuries like cuts or scrapes, and post-surgical inflammation. Curcumin has no toxic effects to humans, so that means no prescription is needed.

Curcumin is able to reduce inflammation because it lowers histamine levels and stimulates the adrenal glands so that it will produce cortisone, which is your own natural painkiller. This can help to alleviate pain from:

- Ulcers – this only induces half the effect of OTC antacids, but it is a cheaper option. It also helps to work against *Helicobacter pylori*, which is the main cause of gastric ulcers.

- Gout

- Osteoarthritis – which is due to the mechanical wear and tear of the joints, such as the shoulder.

- Backache – this is caused by muscular pulls, strain, or sprains.

- Headache

- Kidney stones and gallstones – it works by thinning the bile and lowering stone formation or dissolving the already formed stone.

- Fibromyalgia

- Diverticulitis – this works by reducing the swelling of the colon pockets.

- Carpal tunnel syndrome

- Rheumatoid arthritis – this is caused by autoimmune dysfunction

There are also several other healing uses for turmeric.

- Mental decline – curcumin is able to bind with heavy metals like lead and cadmium, which reduces the toxicity of these heavy metals and protect the brain.

- Atherosclerosis – it is able to reduce the formation of blood clumps.

- Warts – it has proven to be active against the papillomavirus.

- Psoriasis – it helps to regulate inflammatory proteins that the immune system secretes; can be applied topically.

- Indigestion

- Viral infections

- Fungal infections – curcumin has at least 20 fungicidal compounds.

- Diabetes – it helps to increase insulin production and lowers blood sugar.

- Depression – it works similar to serotonin.

How Much to Take

Typically, you can take two tablespoons and mix it into the water to form a paste to use for topical applications, like arthritic joints or wounds. Internally, you can take a half to one and a half teaspoons of dried root powder each day. This would be 250 milligrams each day in the form of a supplement, or 400 to 600 milligrams of turmeric extract in a supplement for no more than three times a day for extreme pain.

It's a good idea to find a supplement that has black

pepper in it as well, or you can add it in when cooking. Adding black pepper to your topical treatments for pain is extremely helpful.

If you plan on taking supplements for your pain, try to find those that are standardized to 95 percent curcuminoids, phospholipid-bound, and containing lecithin.

Adding turmeric to your regular diet is a great way to help prevent disease and pain. Ayurvedic medicine uses a lot of turmeric. Ayurvedic medicine is the traditional Indian healing practice. Here are some great ways to add turmeric to your diet:

- Use it for what it is, a spice, in main dishes like soups, beans, vegetables, rice, turkey, and chicken.

- Mix it into salad dressings, sautéed onions, eggs, bone broth, smoothies, potatoes, glazes, and marinades.

- Curry paste can be purchased, or you could make your own and mix it into soups or stir-fries.

- Add some onto cruciferous vegetables like kale, brussels sprouts, broccoli, cauliflower. The phenethyl isothiocyanates that the crucifers contain combine with curcumin to reduce your risk of prostate tumors.

- Adding in black pepper helps to improve the bioavailability of curcumin.

- Turmeric tea or golden milk is also a great option.

There are over 7000 studies that have found that turmeric can help beat all types of pain, including back, neck, and shoulder pains.

Ginger

Do you have ginger in your spice rack? Maybe you need to move it to your medicine cabinet. Besides the fact that it is a tasty spice, which is often used in holiday treats, ginger is able to diminish nausea and soothe upset stomachs, and studies have found that it can help ease inflammation and pain.

All through history, ginger has been a common treatment for digestive problems and nausea. Now science has found that it is also beneficial for those with chronic pain like arthritis.

In fact, a study at the University of Miami found that ginger extract could end up being a substitute for nonsteroidal anti-inflammatory drugs. Their study examined 247 patients and the effects of highly concentrated ginger extract to osteoarthritis of the knee. The ginger was able to reduce the stiffness and pain in the joints by 40% over the placebo.

During the six-week double-blind study, the participants were given either a highly concentrated ginger extract made from *Alpinia galangal* and *Zingiber officinale* or a placebo.

Beneficial Properties

Why is ginger so amazing? Ginger has antioxidant, anti-inflammatory, and anti-ulcer properties, and they have a small amount of analgesic property.

Research studies have found that the benefits of ginger come from several different compounds, which includes shogaols and gingerols. All of these compounds have anti-oxidant and anti-inflammatory properties. Besides being helpful for treating arthritis, ginger is also great for treating heart or digestive conditions and even cancer.

Its anti-inflammatory agents help get rid of pain and improve arthritis symptoms. Ginger's compounds work like COX-2 inhibitors, in the same way as traditional medications for psoriatic arthritis and rheumatoid arthritis.

The University of Georgia did another study built on previous work that identified ginger's success as an anti-inflammatory agent in rodents. A professor from the kinesiology department, Patrick O'Connor, led two studies that looked at how heat-treated and raw ginger affected muscle pain. The 74 participants consumed either heat-treated or raw ginger over an 11-day period and then took part in moderately tax arm exercises.

The effects were amazing. The ginger reduced the pain in both groups of participants by more than 25%, with both types of ginger providing nearly the exact same results. O'Connor said that this kind of exercise-induced pain is a very common pain across all activities. Ginger is able to help reduce this type of pain by reducing the inflammation in the muscle.

Osteoarthritis, which is a common cause of chronic shoulder, back, and neck pain, is one of the most common forms of arthritis and nearly 20 to 27 million people in the US suffer from it. This wear-and-tear condition tends to affect the larger, weight-bearing joints.

The majority of the studies on the anti-inflammatory and anti-oxidant properties of ginger have mainly been studied in rodents, but across everything, the results have shown a strong potential for human pain relief. There was one study that discovered that fresh ginger had good potential for anti-oxidant properties that were healing and protective when it came to cellular stress.

As far as its anti-inflammatory effects, studies have found that the different compounds found in ginger are able to help with pain in a variety of ways. One particular study found that ginger extract was able to reduce the elevated expression of TNF-a and NFkB in rats with liver cancer. Elevated levels of these compounds are typically linked to inflammatory diseases such as arthritis, diabetes, Crohn's, asthma, allergy, and cardiovascular disease.

Even though there aren't a lot of human research and trials, it does look as if ginger is able to help with pain specifically as it relates to inflammation.

Adding Ginger to Your Diet

Picking the best form of ginger is probably one of the biggest challenges to reaping its reward. You can get ginger in oils, powders, teas, tinctures, capsules, and foods made from the fresh or dried roots of the ginger plant.

Experts say that the best way to reap the benefits of ginger is to consume it in a 100 to 225 mg supplement. Make sure that you talk to your doctor first before you add this supplement to your diet. Ginger can interfere with blood-thinning medications such as warfarin. When picking out a supplement, try to find brands that use the words "super-critical extraction," because it provides you with the purest ginger and the best effect. It's best if you take your supplement along with food because too much ginger on an empty stomach can upset it.

While they smell great, foods such as ginger tea, gingerbread, and gingersnaps might not contain enough ginger to receive the needed benefits. Once your doctor says it's okay to try a ginger supplement, start out with 100 to 200 mg capsules, taking one a day for four to six weeks to see how strong dosage you need.

If you like to have that tangy zip of fresh ginger, I've got great news. Georgia State College & University in Milledgeville and the University of Georgia in Athens found that just a few added tablespoons of fresh ginger are able to ease exercise muscle pain.

Mix a few tablespoons into your food by grating the ginger into a stir-fry or over a salad. You can also grate some into a pot of hot water and let it steep for five minutes to make a soothing tea.

Before Using Ginger

While ginger is a lot safer to use than prescription strength painkillers, it can create problems with certain medications. Here are four things to remember before you start supplementing ginger.

1. Check in with your doctor.

Before you start to add in a significant amount of ginger to your diet, speak with your doctor about any of the possible issues, which include drug interactions. This is extremely important for people who take Coumadin because ginger can reverse the effects of the drug.

2. Pick the correct formulation

After you have spoken with your doctor, this probably is the most important part. As stated earlier, supplements are probably the best way to go. While many of the other options in this book work best when rub onto the skin in a tincture or cream form, ginger works best from the inside out. Follow the instructions from earlier to figure out the dosage you need. Keep in mind that 225 mg of ginger is almost equivalent to a bushel of fresh ginger, so that would be quite hard to eat in a single day.

3. Dose correctly.

Your doctor can also help you to pick the right dosage for you if you're not interested in playing the guessing game. Your doctor will start you out with 100 mg of ginger each day and test up to 200 mg for four to six weeks. You will have to keep track of any changes in your pain levels and your mobility.

4. Incorporate ginger into your life.

Whether you're supplementing with ginger or not, you can add more ginger into your daily life in many different forms. Keep some ginger root on hand and add to foods. Ginger freezes well, so keep some peeled ginger in your freezer and cut of one-inch squares and add to boiling water to create a tea.

Select, Prepare, and Store

When you buy ginger in the grocery store, it is likely ten months old. The skin is darker, and a little tough, and the inside is dark yellow. In some mature ginger, there can be a blue streak running through it. This ginger is Hawaiian blue ring ginger and is typically only available between December and April. This is a very pungent and juicy ginger.

Young ginger has a thinner skin that you won't have to peel before you use it. The flesh of the ginger is less fibrous and tough, which is the reason why it is the best ginger for creating that pile of pink ginger that comes along with sushi.

When you see a large knot of ginger, this is referred to as a hand. Try to find a firm and unwrinkled hand that doesn't have any signs of mold. If you are only looking for a small piece, it is okay to break off what you need. There are some Chinese medicine practitioners that believe that the best piece of ginger for medicinal use is a piece that is shaped like a person.

Whether you purchase a small piece or a large one

that looks like a mini person, you can store ginger in the refrigerator packed in a loosely wrapped paper towel in a sealed plastic container. You can also freeze ginger in a plastic container. The best thing about freezing is that it can be grated more easily. Ginger can last for several weeks when stored in the fridge, and several months when frozen.

Make sure you peel the ginger before you store it. This can be done easily and safely with a spoon.

Devil's Claw

A lot of people who suffer from arthritis, as well as other types of back or joint pain, are turning to Devil's claw for help. Devil's claw is probably the most common home remedy for pain. But Devil's claw doesn't just help with pain. Much like turmeric, Devil's claw is a natural anti-inflammatory. Devil's claw is used like the South American cat's claw root to treat digestive problems and arthritis.

It tends to also be used along with bromelain to help relieve different types of joint pain, especially when it is caused by arthritis.

Devil's claw can provide many other health benefits other than pain relief. There is even one report that has studied its possibility of anticancer potential.

To fully understand what Devil's claw does, you need to understand what it is. Devil's claw is the *Harpogophytum procumbens* plant, which is a plant that is located in the Kalahari savanna of Southern Africa, Namibian steppes, and Madagascar.

Supplements of Devil's claw are typically made up of its dried roots. European and African folk and traditional medical practitioners have given attention to Devil's claw for more than 100 years to help with some pregnancy symptoms, relieve pain, reduce fever, and digestive ills.

It's believed that Devil's claw's benefits come from its content of iridoid glucosides, including harpagoside. These iridoids work as anti-inflammatories that are commonly found in plants and bind with glucose molecules. This is the reason why the compounds are known as iridoid glucosides. The European Scientific Cooperative on Phytotherapy says that Devil's claw contains at least 1% harpagoside.

Devil's claw also has phytosterols and bioflavonoids, which are plant-based antioxidants that have antispasmodic properties. These are helpful for treating digestive problems.

France even allowed marketing for Devil's claw claiming that it is "traditionally used for symptomatic relief of painful joint disorders." ESCOP has approved the use of Devil's claw for dyspepsia, loss of appetite, tendonitis, and painful arthritis.

In Greek, *Harpagophytum* translates to "hook plant." Growing originally and predominantly in Africa, the plant appears like it is covered with hooks. These hooks protect the fruit that grows on the plant, which allows it to be able to attach to the fur of animals to help spread its seeds.

There are several different uses for Devil's claw, which include reducing headache, back and chest pain, soothing heartburn, relieving the symptoms of gout, and boosting heart health.

Western medicine was introduced to the powers of Devil's claw root by South African farmer, G.H. Mehnert, who noticed how the natives use the plant. The first use of the plant in Europe was in 1953, where they used it for allergies, bladder, kidney, bile, liver, and arthritic complaints.

There was one study performed on Devil's claw where patients suffered from slight to moderate muscular tension, or slight muscular pain in the neck, back and shoulder. Using a double-blind, randomized basis, 31 participants were given doses of the extract of Devil's claw two times a day, and another 32 participants were given a placebo. The therapy lasted for four weeks. They achieved a highly significant clinical efficacy in cases of slight to moderate muscular pain.

Using Devil's Claw and Side Effects

Devil's claw can be used as a tea or in pill form. To get the benefits of Devil's claw, the plant's root is dried and packed into a tablet or capsule. It can also be used to make a liquid extract or an ointment to rub onto the skin. If you want to make a tea, you can brew four to five grams of the root in a cup of hot water. Drink this once a day for relief from muscle and joint pain.

If you want to take a supplement, try to find a product that contains extracts of Devil's claw with a standard of two to three percent iridoid glycosides. Make sure that the supplement comes from a safe company with a proven track record, and they list all ingredients and facts. Depending on the intensity of your pain, you can take 200 to 2500 mg each day. Start with 200 and increase the dosage until you receive relief from pain. Make sure you take a dosage for at least a week before increasing it.

There isn't much information as to the possible side effects. There are some sources that suggest that you shouldn't take it if you're breastfeeding or pregnant because they don't know what could happen.

WebMD says that people who have a peptic ulcer, gallstones, diabetes, low blood pressure, hypertension, or heart problems should steer clear from Devil's claw. There is a little bit of evidence that could suggest that it can affect these conditions. This means that if you suffer from one or more of these conditions, you should make sure to speak with health care provider and stay closely monitored.

There are some medications that might interact with Devil's claw. This includes medications that affect the liver because Devil's claw can slow down the liver's breakdown of the drugs. Warfarin is one such drug that could be affected by Devil's claw.

Other Benefits

1. Arthritis Relief

Curing osteoarthritis symptoms have been the most studied use of Devil's claw. A Japanese study performed in 2010 found that Devil's claw was able to reduce inflammation due to arthritis in mice.

Overall, Devil's claw is virtually accepted by the majority of doctors as a "supportive treatment for degenerative, painful rheumatism." Rheumatic diseases are marked by chronic inflammation and are typically located in the joint, fibrous, and muscle tissue pain.

When Devil's claw was tested on different rheumatic disorders, there was a significant reduction of pain in the back, knee, hip, shoulder, elbow, wrist, and hand. The same study also found that the patient's quality of life was improved. In fact, 60 % of participants ended up being able to reduce or quit using their pain medication.

Besides reducing pain, Devil's claw could possibly help prevent bone loss. The majority of tests have only been performed in labs on animals, but there are still lots of promising signs that the plant can prevent bone loss in inflammatory osteoporosis.

2. Weight Loss

The anti-inflammatory root could be able to help you lose weight. An Irish study discovered that Devil's claw was able to stop or slow down the production of ghrelin, which is the hunger hormone. By lowering hunger pangs, people who suffer from overeating issues could find that their appetites are lowered to average, which will aid in weight loss.

It could also end up helping to prevent weight-related atherosclerosis through the way that it is able to suppress inflammation.

3. Natural Painkiller

The pain benefits don't just work for arthritis pain. Even though they don't quite understand why, Devil's claw is able to reduce inflammation and the pain that it causes in several different conditions, including pain that is acute.

Some sources have also stated that Devil's claw is a great medication for sciatica. It's important to know, though, that there haven't been any studies performed on its effects on sciatica.

4. Fight's Chronic Inflammation

The most valuable part of Devil's claw is how it is able to lower inflammation throughout the body, which is one of the main causes of most diseases. Some of the most recent research has been able to find that Devil's claw is able to inhibit TBF-a, which is a cytokine that is a part of the regular inflammation response that happens throughout the body as it works to regulate your immune system.

This is a very important part of the body because whenever TNF-a is working harder than it should be, chronic inflammation will end up happening, which can then end up leading to several different types of diseases. The majority of studies aiming to prevent inflammatory diseases like IBD, psoriatic arthritis, psoriasis, and rheumatic diseases tries to determine how to inhibit TNF-a.

Cloves

When a person hears the word clove, they are often thinking about garlic cloves. Much like garlic, which we will talk about next, the health benefits of the herb clove dates back to over 2000 years. They are pretty amazing.

In tropical climates, cloves are typically harvested by hand, and it comes from the cute little unopened pink flower buds that grow on the evergreen clove tree. It looks similar to little pretzel sticks or even tiny nails.

Its hard exterior helps to protect the active elements in cloves, which is the light-yellow oil called eugenol, which is what contributes the majority of its health benefits and makes it a natural anti-inflammatory.

After it received a write up in the *New York Times*, cloves gained in popularity as a health item. The article stated that a common health benefit of using clove oil was as a safe and natural alternative of the more commonly used analgesics that contained benzocaine for toothaches.

A gel that was clove-based work just as well as benzocaine for treating patients who received needle stick on both sides of the gums five times over a ten-minute period as compared to people who received a placebo.

These findings were right on track with the use of eugenol extracts used in American dentistry and OTC mouthwashes, throat sprays, and toothpaste.

A study recently done by Miguel Hernandez University went straight to the biggest benefit of cloves. The researchers found that cloves were the top natural antioxidant spice that can and should be used in the food industry because of its natural high levels of phenolic compounds, as well as its antioxidant capacity.

Experts also consider cloves to be a nutrient-dense spice. Two ounces of cloves have 63 % of the daily value of manganese that humans need, along with vitamin C, dietary fiber, vitamin K, and omega-3 fatty acids.

Since cloves are so nutrient dense, cloves have been given the best score in the Oxygen Radical Absorption Capacity that was created by Tufts University for the USDA.

A single drop of clove essential oil can provide you with 400 times more antioxidants per unit volume than the magical goji berries. You can look at a 15-milliliter bottle of clove essential oil and compare it to the antioxidant power of 40 quarts of blueberries.

Clove is often used as an expectorant and used to treat an upset stomach. Clove oil is also great for bad bread, diarrhea, and hernia. Cloves can also be used to help with vomiting, nausea, and gas.

Clove is also often used on the skin to help ease pain and can be used for throat and mouth inflammation. When it comes to manufacturing, clove is often used in cigarettes, perfumes, cosmetics, soaps, and toothpaste.

Early research has found that applying a gel that contains ground cloves for five minutes before being struck by a needle is able to reduce the pain from the stick, similar to benzocaine.

Safety of Cloves

Used as a food additive, clove is safe for the majority of people to take by mouth. There isn't enough information about its safety when the clove is taken in a large medicinal amount.

It is perfectly safe to use cream or oil that contains clove when applied to the skin. However, repeated and frequent applications of clove oil on the gums or in the mouth can cause damage to the mucous membranes, skin, tooth pulp, and gums.

Children should not take clove oil by mouth. It can cause severe side effects like fluid imbalances, liver damage, and seizures. It should be safe to consume food containing cloves when pregnant or breastfeeding. Medicinal amounts of clove have not been studied, so if you are pregnant or breastfeeding, stay safe, and avoid medicinal doses.

Some anticoagulant drugs can be affected by cloves. Cloves can slow down clotting, so be careful.

Using Cloves

Cloves are typically taken in supplement form. The most common form of cloves is the essential oil. You can also add cloves to recipes to add flavor and health benefits.

When using clove oil, make sure that you dilute the oil in a carrier oil. Full strength could end up irritating your skin.

Garlic

There is a theoretical benefit of garlic, and that is arthritis and pain relief when consumed orally. There are also several other ways that you can take garlic. Garlic can be eaten cooked or raw. You can also find it in dried or powdered form, as well as in tablets or capsules. You can also find garlic in liquid extracts and in oils. It's important that you speak with your doctor before you start to take a garlic supplement for a natural pain remedy.

Garlic contains anti-inflammatory and antioxidant properties that are able to help ease the pain from arthritis and other types of joint pain. There was a study published in the *Soviet Archives of Internal Medicine* in 1999 that stated that garlic taken twice a day for four to six weeks was able to work just as well for rheumatoid arthritis as conventional therapy. However, not every single study on the use of garlic for pain provides positive results. For example, if you take garlic for leg pain during walking that is caused by poor circulation due to peripheral arterial disease, you probably won't reap any benefits.

Another great attribute of garlic is that it is able to increase the potency of nonsteroidal anti-inflammatory drugs that you take to help with pain. This means that you will receive an even greater relief from pain. However, if you want to try this, make sure that you talk to your doctor first. Garlic is also able to add to the effects of other drugs. For example, garlic is also able to magnify the effects of blood-thinning drugs such as warfarin and aspirin. Garlic oil is also able to decrease how fast the liver is able to break down certain types of medications. This can end up increasing the medications effects and side effects. Some examples include chlorzoxazone, acetaminophen, and theophylline, and even drugs that are used for anesthesia during surgery such as isoflurane and halothane.

The selenium content of garlic is what makes it helpful for managing arthritis pain or even preventing arthritis. Garlic contains novel sulfur compounds, one such compound is called thiacremonone. This is able to help inhibit your body's inflammatory responses, which means it is a useful agent when it comes to treating inflammatory and arthritic diseases.

The antioxidant content of garlic is also able to reduce inflammation, and thus it will help to manage pain. Antioxidant nutrients are able to help reduce the inflammatory symptoms that come along with inflammatory joint diseases.

Amazing Facts

The following facts came from the University of Maryland Medical Center, *Journal of Immunology Research*, and *Journal of Immunology*.

- All plants that come from the genus Allium are known for producing organic sulfur compounds, which contain interesting pharmacological and biological properties. Garlic is among this group, *Allium sativum*, which is the most widely used.

- When they are isolated and extracted, these compounds exhibit a large spectrum of healthful effects that fight against microbial infections, which are also used to help protect against heart disease.

- Currently, they are looking at how garlic can

help to boost the immune system, and even fight cancer.

- One of garlic's potent sulfur-based compounds is allicin, which is responsible for the smell of garlic but is probably also the reason for its antibacterial properties.

Benefits

People will often refer to garlic as the "stinking rose," but it does seem to have a full bouquet of benefits. But it also matters how you prepare it. Research has found that if you heat garlic too soon, it will interfere with the health benefits that come from allicin.

This means that if you have crushed, minced, or chopped garlic, allow it to sit for five to ten minutes before you cook it. If you can't wait, and you go ahead and throw it into some hot oil or boiling water, all you are doing is deactivating its beneficial enzyme. Patience is most definitely a virtue when you are preparing this golden nugget.

Another great thing about garlic is that it is cheap. A head of garlic isn't that expensive, and you can even sometimes find them in groups of three. You can also buy an expensive jar of pre-chopped garlic, which equals several cloves. This means that it is a cheap option for pain relief.

To take your garlic, you have several options. One way to consume your garlic is to eat a clove every morning. Some people will finely chop or grate it, allow it to rest for five to ten minutes, and then mix it into water and drink it. You can also incorporate more garlic into your cooking. It's best to aim for two to three cloves of fresh garlic every day to help treat your shoulder, neck, or back pain. Most websites will recommend you consume them first thing in the morning, but you can also mix them into your foods so that it's not so strong. Just make sure you let it rest before you cook it.

Another way to get pain relief from garlic is through a garlic oil rub. This works as a topical analgesic. Place ten whole cloves of garlic in two ounces of sesame or coconut oil. Allow the oil to heat and cook the garlic until they turn brown. Strain the garlic cloves out of the oil and store the oil in a small glass jar. Make sure you use the oil within the next few days.

If you want to take a supplement, you can find supplements that range from 150 mg to 2400 mg. You will have to test to see which strength works best for your pain level.

Safety

It appears that garlic is safe for the majority of adults, but it is best if you talk to your doctor before taking a supplement, especially if you are currently on any medicine or have a health condition. Garlic can even interfere with the effectiveness of the drug saquinavir, an HIV drug. Some possible side effects could include allergic reactions, an upset stomach, body and breath odor, and heartburn. If you already have a bleeding disorder, garlic may make it worse because of the blood-thinning properties. If you have planned surgery or dental work, you need to use garlic with caution.

Marjoram

When people use marjoram for pain, they use its essential oil. Sweet marjoram oil is created from the steam distillation of the tops of the plant, and it is a cousin of oregano. The resulting yellow-green essential oil has a camphoraceous, woody, spicy, and warm scent that will remind you of cardamom and nutmeg.

Meanwhile, you also have Spanish marjoram oil, which is a different essential oil that comes from marjoram plants, and it has a red-orange hue. This marjoram was originally native to the Mediterranean areas and North America, today it is widely grown for large-scale commercial use of its oil in Spain, Tunisia, Germany, France, Egypt, and, recently, the United States.

According to folklore, the Egyptians would dedicate the marjoram plant to Osiris, the god of the underworld. They used it to produce love potions, unguents, and medicines. The Romans and Greeks consider this herb to be an herb of happiness and they offered it to the goddess of beauty, love, and fertility, Aphrodite.

In the culinary world, sweet marjoram is an excellent way to add flavor to salads, soups, and other delicious dishes.

Marjoram tea is also popular among women to help promote a better flow of breast milk and ease menopausal symptoms. Sweet marjoram oil will also provide you with positive effects when used in:

- Topical applications as lotion, salve, or cream.

- Massage therapy when it is mixed in with a mild carrier oil or added to bath water.

- Vapor therapy through vaporizers and burners,

When it is used as an inhalant or with aromatherapy, sweet marjoram oil works great for people with insomnia and can't settle down for bed.

Composition

The main chemical make-up of sweet marjoram oil is y-terpineol, terpinene-4-ol, linalyl acetate, cissabinene hydrate, Linalool, terpinolene, p-cymene, y-terpinene, a-terpinene, and sabinene. The oil mixes perfectly with tea tree, eucalyptus, bergamot, chamomile, cedarwood, cypress, and lavender.

How it Works

There are lots of different health benefits that you can get from marjoram, but since we are focusing on pain, here is how it helps different types of pain:

- Analgesic – it helps to alleviate pain related to headache, toothache, inflammation, fevers, and colds.

- Emmenagogue – it helps to regulate painful and irregular menstrual periods.

Safety and Side Effects

If used appropriately, sweet marjoram is perfectly safe. However, it is best if you don't use it, or pretty much any essential oil, if you have an existing condition, or if you are breastfeeding or pregnant. Since it does have emmenagogue properties, which stimulates blood flow, you should never use sweet marjoram oil during pregnancy.

Sweet marjoram oil can also cause allergic reactions or hypersensitivity, so make sure you perform a patch test on a small area of skin to see how you could react to it when used topically. If you mix it with a mild carrier oil, it will help lessen its sensitizing effect.

How to Use

There are several different ways to use marjoram to relieve pain. The essential oil makes it extremely easy as well because you can add some to baths or massages for soothing effects. For a more specific pain like neck, back, or shoulder, dilute some marjoram oil into a cream. Rub the cream onto the painful area, and you will experience some relief.

Parsley

You are probably familiar with parsley as a fresh herb or dried spice, but it has also been proven to be amazing for your health. Even if you only eat parsley in a small amount, there are loads of health benefits because it is full of beneficial nutrients, antioxidants, and essential oil, so much that it is often referred to as a superfood.

It is derived from the Petroselinum plant. Parsley and its oil have been used as a natural anti-inflammatory, antiseptic, diuretic, and detox remedy for centuries. Today, many research studies have started to back up health claims that everybody else has believed for years.

In the *Journal of Traditional Chinese Medicine*, a study was published in 2013 that said parsley has been used to help treat various dermal diseases, diabetes, urinary disease, cardiac disease, hypertension, and gastrointestinal disorder.

The amazing benefits of parsley come from its active

ingredient, which includes nutrients such as vitamins A, K, and C, essential oils such as apiol and myristicin, antioxidant flavonoids, and phenolic compounds.

This means that parsley is an all-natural and safe plant that you can add to your diet so that you can reap its digestion, antifungal, antibacterial, antidiabetic, brain protector, heart protector, and radical scavenger benefits.

Even though there is still more formal research needed, there is already strong evidence associated with parsley's ability to fight the following disorders and symptoms:

- Skin problems

- Poor immunity

- Constipation

- Acid reflux

- Gas

- Edema or bloating

- Arthritis

- Bad breath

- Kidney stones

- Digestive problems

- Bladder infection

- Anemia

- Oxidative stress or free radical damage

- Inflammation

- Pain relief

Parsley has been used for decades to help relieve pain associated with arthritis and other joint diseases. It is packed full of vitamin K, magnesium, and calcium, which all help to reduce the inflammation that causes pain.

Consuming parsley also leads to faster excretion of uric acid. This will end up leading to less joint stiffness and swelling that is associated with uric acid. It is also a great cure for osteoarthritis because it promotes bone health. It contains folate and calcium, which helps to protect the bone from wearing down.

Consuming Parsley

It is believed that drinking parsley tea throughout the day will help improve your joint range of motion. Here is a great recipe for parsley tea:

- Boil eight ounces of water.

- Rinse off a quarter cup of fresh parsley leaves in cool water.

- Pat them dry and roughly chop them. You can also leave them whole, but chopping will release some of the oil, which makes the tea stronger.

- Add the leaves to a cup and cover with the boiling water.

- Steep for ten minutes and then strain out the leaves.

- Sweeten with a bit of honey if needed, and enjoy.

You should try to drink half a cup of tea before breakfast and then another half before dinner. If you have a flare up of pain, you can drink another half cup.

Any unused tea can be refrigerated for later use. This tea is a great way to receive several different minerals and vitamins.

You don't just have to consume parsley in tea form. It is a delicious herb to add to different types of foods. There are also several different varieties of parsley out there. Italian flat leaf is fragrant, while curly parsley is a little more bitter. There are several other types as well, way too many to list. Parsley is a very versatile herb to cook.

Italian flat leaf parsley is great for salads and sauces. Curly leaf parsley is great for seasonings on chicken and beef.

Rosemary

A popular essential oil that is being used today is extracted from the *Rosmarinus officinalis* plant. This plant is very well known throughout the Mediterranean for its herbal and culinary benefits. It has been used for many health purposes.

Rosemary is related to mint but looks a lot like lavender. Its leaves look like flat pine needles that have been brushed with silver. It has a woodsy, citrusy fragrance that has become popular in many apothecaries, gardens, and kitchens all over the world. It got its name from the Latin words "ros" meaning dew and "marinus" meaning sea or simply "dew of the sea."

An old legend states that the Virgin Mary placed her blue wrap over a rosemary bush while she took a rest. The white flowers then turned blue. The bush then became known as the "Rose of Mary."

Rosemary is sacred to the Romans, Greeks, Hebrews, and Egyptians. It was used as protection against plagues and to scare off evil spirits. Rosemary essential oil is clear with a refreshing herbal smell. It can be a bit watery. Essential oils are made from the fresh flowers by using steam. It will yield one to two percent.

Paracelsus, a German-Swiss physician, loved its health benefits. During the 1500s he helped people understand the benefits of herbal medicine. He loved rosemary oil due to its ability to strengthen the whole body. It could help heal organs such as the brain, heart, and liver.

Uses

Rosemary can be used as salad dressings along with thousands of other uses. It is very hardy and will grow very easy either inside or out. Add a whole sprig to soups for a one of a kind flavor. High-quality rosemary oil has expectorant, antioxidant, anti-inflammatory, anti-infection, antifungal, anticatarrhal, anticancer, antibacterial, and analgesic properties.

Here is a list of some health problems that rosemary oil can help you with:

- Clarity – Place a few drops in your hands, rub them together to warm up the oil. Cup your hands over your nose and mouth for about one minute.

- Cough – Massage a couple drops over the throat and chest every couple of hours.

- Headaches – Place a few drops in your hands. Cup your hands over your nose and mouth for a minute. You could also apply a few drops topically to the part of your head that hurts.

- Memory and Learning – Diffuse the oils in the rooms you are occupying. Take a few whiffs straight from the bottle. Rub some on your temples. Apply to your toes every day.

- Vaginal Infections – Massage a few drops in and around the vaginal area. Test the area for sensitivity before you place it inside the vagina.

Rosemary teas and oils can be added to lotions and shampoos. By using the oil daily, it can help to stimulate the hair follicles. This will help with growing long, strong, and luscious hair. You could also massage the oil into your scalp to remove dandruff and nourish it.

You can also use rosemary oil on pets to help with hair growth. It will help their coats become shiny. It also helps to fight fungal infections in their ears.

Rosemary oil is a natural disinfectant and can be used as a mouthwash to help prevent bad breath. By getting rid of the bacteria in the mouth, it can prevent cavities, the build-up of plaque, and other dental problems. Rosemary has a mesmerizing aroma that makes it a wonderful inhalant.

Rosemary oil can be put into cosmetics, fresheners, bath oils, perfumes, and candles. It will give your mind and energy boost when inhaled. When diluted 50/50, you can apply rosemary oil to wrists and ankles, vitaflex and chakra points, inhaled, diffuse, or as a supplement.

Benefits

Rosemary oil has been studied and used since ancient times for many health benefits. It is still used today for the same purposes. These include the following:

- Indigestion – Rosemary oil can be used to relieve bloating, constipation, stomach cramps, and flatulence. It can be helpful to stimulate appetite. Researchers show that it can detoxify the liver. It can regulate how the liver creates and releases bile. This is the main part of our digestive process.

- Stress Relief – Rosemary can decrease the level of cortisol. This is the hormone the body releases in the salivary gland during the flight-or-fight process. One study shows that inhaling lavender and rosemary oils for about five minutes can reduce cortisol levels significantly. This decreases the dangers of chronic stress.

- Pain Relief – Rosemary oil has been widely known for its pain-relieving properties. It is used to treat arthritis, muscle pain, and headaches. Massage some oil onto the affected area. You could add it to hot bath water to help treat rheumatism. Its anti-inflammatory properties surely help to relieve pain from joint aches and sprains.

- Boost the Immune System – Studies show that inhaling the essential oil while massaging it into the affected area can increase free radical's scavenging activities. Antioxidants are needed to fight disease and infection. By inhaling or using rosemary oil regularly, it can give your immunity a boost to help you fight off diseases caused by free radicals.

- Respiratory problems – Inhaling rosemary oil can relieve and treat respiratory problems like the flu, sore throat, colds, allergies, and throat congestion. Because of its antiseptic properties, rosemary oil can be used to fight respiratory infections. Due to its antispasmodic properties, it can help treat bronchial asthma with specific treatment programs.

Rosemary oil does great things for anxiety. Using sachets that contain rosemary and lavender essential oils can reduce anxiety caused by taking tests.

Using rosemary can help brain health. Rosemary can

help improve the moods of healthy adults. A study done over a month's time using aromatherapy that included orange, lavender, lemon, and rosemary oils increased the cognitive functions of Alzheimer's patients.

Making Infused Oil

Rosemary essential oil is so versatile that it's so easy to use in aromatherapy with many different aromas. It can blend well with peppermint, chamomile, lemongrass, citronella, thyme, basil, sage, clary, frankincense, and lavender.

It is easy to make your own rosemary oil by putting a couple sprigs of totally dry rosemary into a glass jar. Fill the jar with olive oil. Put the lid on the jar and give it a slight shake. Store the jar in a dark, warm place for two weeks. Remove the rosemary sprigs. Keep the oil stored in the glass jar. For a fragrant bath, add ¼ cup to a tub of hot water. Blend with some balsamic vinegar for a tasty salad dressing.

How it Works

To help relieve congestion in the respiratory tract, pain, mental fatigue, and help blood circulation, use rosemary oil in vaporizers, burners, in a relaxing bath, or just massage it into the affected areas. To use as a hair and skin care agent, use blended oils in shampoos, conditioners, lotions, or creams. You only need to add about three drops of essential oil to a bath.

Safe?

Rosemary oil is an effective and safe oil that is good for a variety of purposes and uses. Before putting it directly onto your skin, dilute it with a carrier oil so it won't cause skin sensitivity. Always do a patch test first.

Breastfeeding or pregnant women should not use rosemary essential oils during pregnancy or while breastfeeding. Always talk to your doctor before giving rosemary oil to children. Never self-treat any chronic disease like Alzheimer's or depression with rosemary oil. This could cause serious problems if you haven't consulted your doctor first.

Side Effects

Sometimes rosemary might cause an allergic reaction. As said above, always talk to your doctor for proper usage. Due to the fact that it is volatile in nature, it could cause spasms and vomiting. Never ingest the essential oil. Again, pregnant women should never use rosemary essential oil as it can cause the miscarriage of an unborn child.

Thyme

For many years thyme has been used in many culinary dishes. It used to be used as a medicine by early Europeans. It was used to treat many different health problems.

Many people use thyme in puns, but nobody really knows where it originated. It is thought to have come from the ancient Greek word "thumus" that means courage. Other people think it came from the Egyptian word "tham" that means courage. Each one of these interpretations shows the main qualities of the herb.

Thyme is a short shrub that originates from the southern part of Europe. It has the smallest leaves of any shrub in a garden. Even though it is small in size, it has always symbolized bravery and strength for thousands of years in many cultures.

From the time of the ancient Greeks, this fragrant herb has been utilized to help overcome adversity and fear. Thyme has been used to help improve courage, overcome shyness, and alleviate depression. People who lived during the Renaissance used to put thyme under their pillow to ward off nightmares. It was also put into coffins to help loved ones enter into the afterlife in Europe.

Cough

Thyme isn't used as a medicine much anymore, but it has several medicinal properties. Other than putting it in your favorite foods, thyme can be used to help with congestion and coughing. Thyme can break up phlegm and will clear the head and chest. For thousands of years, it has been used to relieve the symptoms of influenza and colds. Dioscorides would drink thyme mixed with vinegar and salt to help get rid of phlegm by sending it through the bowels.

Thyme's drying effects make it great for colds and other conditions that cause the lungs to become congested by mucus. Thyme can be used to help control coughing spasms and can be used as an antitussive especially when battling whooping cough.

Scientists have started validating thyme's use in helping cure bronchitis. In a double-blind study, researchers saw that patients who are given dried extracts of thyme mixed with evening primrose had quicker a healing time than patients that were given a placebo.

In another study, researchers found that an extract of thyme mixed with ivy leaves controlled their patient's cough two days faster than patients who took a placebo. This combination is safe for children between the ages of two and 17.

Thyme can be used to help with the symptoms of upper-respiratory infections, whooping cough, and bronchitis. Thyme is one of the ten herbs found in the cough drop Ricola.

Purification

There are several cultures that practice the burning of dried thyme to purify their homes and temples. The fragrance has been described as earthy, bitter, but altogether pleasant.

It was thought that thyme can prevent evil spirits from entering the home or a person. One Roman doctor thought thyme could send away any venomous creatures.

Infection

Thyme contains chemicals called phytochemicals that help the body fight infections. Thyme can kill yeast, fungal, and bacterial infections. It can also kill parasites like roundworm and hookworm. Some herbalists will use thyme and other herbs in a vaginal suppository to help with Group B Streptococcus during the last stages of pregnancy.

Thyme belongs to the mint family and is rich in essential oils. This gives the plant its powerful scent and medicinal powers.

Ancient Sumerians used thyme like an antiseptic. Egyptians mummified their dead using thyme. Roman emperors would chew thyme after a meal thinking it would prevent them from being poisoned. During the Victorian

Age, nurses would disinfect bandages by washing them in thyme water.

Thyme's ability to fight microbes is the main reason it

is used to preserve food and can be used to fight many different types of bacterial infections. You can use it as a wash for minor mouth infections, inflamed gums, or sore gums. Making a gargle with honey that has been infused with thyme can help soothe a sore throat. Listerine has used thyme oil in its mouthwash since 1879 to help kill germs that cause bad breath.

Thyme can inhibit the properties that cause bacterial cells to become resistant to antibiotics. There are an estimated two million people who get antibiotic-resistant infections every year in the United States. These infections could result in over 23,000 deaths. Thyme along with other herbs that have the same properties might be that ray of hope to help with the threat of antibiotic-resistant bacteria.

Digestion

Just like most herbs, thyme tastes amazing but also helps with digestion. It can be eaten in meals to support a healthy digestive system. If needed, it can be taken in bigger amounts to help with flatulence, belching, and bloating. It can help to calm digestive spasms to help with irritable bowel syndrome or diarrhea.

Pain

Most people don't think that a common herb would have the ability to help relieve pain, but thyme has the ability to cure headaches and sciatica. Some people believe that thyme is as good as clove for an oral anesthetic. Thyme oil was used during World War I to help treat wounds.

Researchers continue to uphold thyme's reputation as a pain reliever. One study found that essential oil made from thyme could relieve menstrual cramps just as well as ibuprofen. It actually works better with time. Women in the ibuprofen group said their cramps weren't relieved as well during the second month. The thyme group said the oil gave more pain relief during the second month.

Thyme essential oil can be rubbed on painful joints. Thyme can be used for gout, and normal everyday aches and pains.

Uses

Thyme is a very popular culinary herb since it goes well with almost everything. It can be a bit spicy and bitter, so take it easy. Thyme gives a pleasing flavor and helps with digestion.

You can throw the entire sprig of thyme into whatever you are cooking. Just remember to remove all the stems before serving the dish. You can tie the thyme with some kitchen twine to help you remove the stems faster.

Thyme tea is a great choice when choosing a medicinal tea. Think about this recipe from Hippocrates: Boil two cups of water with three tablespoons of thyme. Cover the pot and let it steep for ten minutes. Drink two glasses each day to help with bronchitis.

Thyme can be prepared as a tea or a tincture which is an alcohol extract. It can also be infused with honey, vinegar, or oil.

You can find thyme essential oil in either white or red. Red is a lot stronger and will cost more. It can also cause skin irritation. The white oil has been refined.

You should use both sparingly but never during pregnancy. To use it topically, dilute it with carrier oil like almond or coconut oil. Do not take thyme essential oil internally if you are not working with a practitioner who is qualified.

The best way to use essential oils is by using a diffuser. Take a whiff when you are in need of some courage.

Here are some dosage suggestions:

Thyme tea: two to six grams of dried tea to one cup boiling water each day.

Thyme Extract: dried thyme in a one to five ratio with 35 % alcohol. Take two to four milliliters three times each day.

Thyme Essential Oil: Dilutions of 1 % or fewer. Place one drop of essential oil to 100 drops of carrier oil.

Special Considerations

Thyme is very safe when used in small quantities.

Pregnant or nursing women shouldn't use thyme or

thyme essential oil. If taken in large dosages, thyme can stimulate menstrual flow or uterine contractions.

Choose thyme due to its chemotype and use it only when diluted and in small amounts. Find an aromatherapist who has been trained on how to use essential oils internally. This will ensure that you take the right amount of this very potent extraction.

Allergic reactions are very rarely reported with thyme usage.

To Sum it up

Thyme is native to the sunny Mediterranean rocky soils. Thyme gives aromatic and powerful medicines in a very small package. Thyme can be eaten regularly in many meals. It can be added to beef dishes, salad dressings, and stews. You can drink tea made from thyme. It can also be made into a tincture. Thyme is great in helping with poor digestion. It also helps with influenza or colds. Research is being done to see how effective thyme can be against antibiotic-resistant bacterial infections.

Conclusion

Thank you for making it through to the end of *Physical Pain Herbal Medicine*, we hope it was informative and was able to provide you with all of the tools you need to achieve your goals whatever they may be.

The next step is to start trying some of these herbal remedies for your pain. Start with one or two and see what works best for you. Make sure that you follow recommended doses; otherwise, you may not get any relief. It's also a good idea to talk to your doctor first to make sure that the source of your pain isn't something major.

Finally, if you found this book useful in any way, a review on Amazon is always appreciated!

Description

Are you tired of dealing with your back, neck, or shoulder pain?

If you answered yes, then you need this book. The power of herbal medicine has been around for centuries, and it's still powerful today.

Prescription medicines and over-the-counter pain killers come with a lot of side effects, and possible addictions. Herbal medicines are a healthier option.

This book has ten herbal remedies that can help reduce pain and inflammation. You will learn about:

- Capsaicin

- Turmeric

- Ginger

- Devil's claw

- Cloves

- Garlic

- Marjoram

- Parsley

- Rosemary

- Thyme

Herbal remedies are a safe and great way to treat ailments without the side effects of Eastern medicine. Get this book today and say goodbye to your pain.

Herbal Medicine Insomnia:

The 10 Best Solutions to Solve Insomnia Naturally

© Copyright 2018 - All rights reserved.

The information in the following pages is broadly considered to be truthful and accurate account of facts, and as such any inattention, use or misuse of the information in question by the reader will render any resulting actions solely under their purview. There are no scenarios in which the publisher or the original author of this work can be in any fashion deemed liable for any hardship or damages that may befall them after undertaking information described herein.

Additionally, the information in the following pages is intended only for informational purposes and should thus be thought of as universal. As befitting its nature, it is presented without assurance regarding its prolonged validity or interim quality. Trademarks that are mentioned are done without written consent and can in no way be considered an endorsement from the trademark holder.

Table of Contents

Introduction

Congratulations on downloading *Herbal Medicine Insomnia: The 10 Best Solutions to Solve Insomnia Naturally* and thank you for doing so.

The following chapters will discuss why insomnia happens in the first place and what are the best natural solutions that there are to combat against it and keep it away for good. Inside this book you will find not only what are the 10 best natural herbs used to overcome insomnia, but several other handy tips as well that you can use for the rest of your life. Herbal teas that help to bring on a good night's sleep will be discussed, as well as why it is a good idea to have certain plant life hanging in the room that you sleep in. You will also get to learn exactly what the circadian clock is and how you can begin to get yours in tune with Mother Nature and her celestial children that are the sun and moon.

The title of the book may say *10 Best solutions*, but more than only 10 tips will be found within its pages.

You will learn about the 10 best herbs to use to defeat insomnia, but plenty of other information that can be used in conjunction with those 10 herbs will be given to you.

There are plenty of books on this subject on the market, thanks again for choosing this one! Every effort was made to ensure it is full of as much useful information as possible, please enjoy!

Chapter 1:

Why Can't You Sleep?

Roughly about 60 million people in the United States suffer from the sleep malady known as insomnia. That is only accounting for one country. Across the entire world insomnia is estimated to disrupt the sleep of about a third of the entire populace. If you were wondering if you were the only one who wasn't capable of getting a solid night's rest, you can be sure that you are not alone.

Insomnia may very well be the oldest of all human conflictions. Since sleeping is as old as mankind, tracing the origins of insomnia back to the original source is an impossible mystery to unravel. Even more, insomnia will most likely never be an affliction that just ups and goes away. As long as there is a human race that needs sleep, there will be insomnia to disrupt it.

Sleep and nature have always shared a very special one of a kind of relationship between each other. The intricate delicacy of this relationship can even be said to be reflective of the process known as evolution and involution. This may sound like a stretch, but the purpose of this book is not just to simply teach you about using different herbs for the sole sake of defeating the cowardly and multifarious, hellish thief of sleep that has been called insomnia. It is much more than that. The purpose of this book is to pull you out of the mundane doldrums that is our modern day rat race of a society and its opulent amount of distractions. The point of this book may be focused on how to use herbs to get better sleep, but that is (like so many things in life) only a thinly veiled simulacrum that is hiding the real truth. The real purpose of this book is to get you back in touch with the glory and splendor that has given birth to every man, woman, child, beast, plant, mineral, grain, atom, and subatomic particle.

The real purpose of this book is to reintroduce you to Mother Nature, for without her constant effort and guidance you would not be here. There would be no planet earth or any other celestial body floating out there in the recess of stellar space. There would be no solar system. There would be no time, space, or time-space. This book would not exist without Mother Nature. No author would have ever constructed a thought to put down in writing. No language would have ever developed. No society would have ever grown out of the mud and waters, later to tower onwards reaching ever closer to the rim of the atmosphere that surrounds our planet. There would be no evolution. There would be no concept of spirit. There would be no sun to wake up to, and no moon to sleep under.

You may think that such an intro is misleading or exaggerated. Well, I would tell you to sleep on it, but we are not there yet. I'm sure that after you put all the information in this book to practical use and you do get some solid sleep, then these words will return to you later and revelation will come. That time has not come yet, though, first you need to learn why insomnia happens in the first place and figure out where something may have gone wrong with your circadian clock. If you are not sure how insomnia may have snuck up on you or are wondering what in the blazes a circadian clock is, then get ready to learn a whole lot more than just that.

Take Sleep Seriously

The average person will, and is supposed to, spend almost have of their lifetime asleep. Reading that may sound factious but if you think about it you will realize it's not. We are up during the daylight hours going to work, being with friends and family, enjoying our hobbies and doing everything that we have to get done before the sun dips away. During those hours we are expending energy and (for many of us) letting our minds run at a frantic pace just to keep up with the current tides. The old axiom of *"There just aren't enough hours in the day."*, is a phrase that many learn to eventually accept as a cold and hard truth. However, there is an ancient trick to reconciling this age-old problem. It is the oldest trick in every book and has been extolled time and time again. The best way to manage your time better during the day, and harness your energy to its fullest potential, is to get a solid 6-8 hours of sleep the night before.

It may be a small tip that you are already aware of, but for the sake of being as comprehensive as possible, you should be getting at least six hours of sleep every night. That is a lowball number, as 8 hours is what just about every medical professional recommends. Even if your schedule doesn't seem to allow it you must make time to receive the proper amount of sleep. If you like to watch television late at night, gallivant around town, or find any other reasons to avoid getting the proper amount of sleep you will have to start altering that before doing anything else. The more sleep you get in the evening, the more hours you have to do what you want the following day. As difficult as this may be to hear, this also applies to business and social engagements. It may seem like the responsible decision is to skip a few hours of sleep, so you can fit more time in to get work done- but it's not. The true responsible decision is to get more and better sleep, so you can work to your fullest ability the following day. This applies to social engagements as well. You may not want to miss out on all the fun or opportunities that seem to come with networking and fraternizing, but if you do not receive the proper amount of sleep then you just won't be your sharpest and most lucid when going to those social engagements. It's a tradeoff that may not seem fair but getting the right amount of sleep is truly the most responsible decision you can make for yourself and those around you.

Sleeping is the most natural way for the body to repair itself. The benefits of getting good sleep cannot be argued. There is a very good reason why doctors often recommend getting plenty of bed rest when someone has a cold or is recovering from an operation. The cells of our bodies repair themselves when we lay down to sleep. A cut on the flesh will not quickly heal unless the body reverts into the "sleep state". When in sleep state, our muscles know it is time to relax and not expend energy, instead harnessing it so it can be utilized the next day. While we are recollecting our energy, maintenance is being performed on those muscles, and our organs as well. The human immune system can become confused when it does not get enough sleep, and when it becomes confused it may not do the work of repairing our bodies the best it should. This is why sleep is something that needs to be taken seriously.

Sleep is not just a necessity for our bodies and cells to repair themselves but is just as important for the mind. We don't just expend physical energy while running around during the day, but mental energy as well. A plethora of thoughts and conflictions, tough decisions and judgment calls, can swell up and leave a festering hive of confusion and stress in our minds. During sleep our minds also have a chance to settle down, turnoff so to speak, and calm down the volatile ocean of scattered thoughts. This is where the phrase, *"Let me sleep on that."*, originates from. It is far easier to make a hard decision after getting a good night's sleep, and also easier to work out the cacophony of stress that has built up during the day.

The human subconscious gets to shine during sleep. Ask any psychologist and they will tell you that the subconscious is not something we can directly interact with on any practical or rationale level. It needs to sort things out for itself without the self-consciousness getting in its way. The only chance it gets to do that and work on its own is while we sleep. The pile of ideas, fears, hopes, and everything else that we encountered and thought of during a normal day would only grow higher and more unstable if not for the subconscious settling things in order while in sleep. This may seem like common knowledge but, before going any further in this book, ask yourself a very important question...

"Do I take sleep seriously enough?"

The reason this question is so important is because, when asking it with astute clarity, you are projecting a direct message to your body, and mind. Since sleeping is not just physical but also mental, creating the right frame of mind before diving into the tips and herbs used to defeat insomnia is paramount. This idea of creating the proper mindset for sleep will be more valuable to some than for others. If your insomnia has been caused due to a purely physical condition, then many of the herbs and tips in this book may be enough to help you. If, however, your insomnia is due to a mental condition then creating the right frame of mind, one that moves you away from insomnia, will be just as important if not more than any advice you will receive here or anywhere else. Thankfully, the herbs you will learn about in this book are all conducive to not just relaxing your tensions and nerves, but also to inducing the proper frame of mind needed to get a good night's rest.

Why Does Insomnia Happen?

One of the biggest problems with trying to combat insomnia is figuring out why you can't fall or stay asleep in the first place. When most people first experience insomnia they don't even realize that they have a problem. They will usually think that it was just one bad day, spiraling into one bad night of (or lack of) sleep and write it off. Then it happens again, and again, until they realize that they have fallen into a very unwanted pattern. It's sad to say, but most people take sleep for granted until they have been bitten by the bug of insomnia. Due to this combination of taking sleep for granted and not noticing that insomnia has happened before it has become a pattern, a large number of people don't ever learn why they became insomniacs in the first place.

One of the most major reasons that insomnia begins is due to medical conditions. If you are positive that your insomnia is because of a medical condition, consult your doctor along with following the guidance of this book. Sometimes the medical condition alone may be causing insomnia, while in other cases it may only be the symptoms of a condition that are causing it. Check the list below to see if your situation matches anything you see.

- Asthma
- Pain in the lower back
- Sinus or nasal allergies
- Arthritis

- Chronic pain (of any sort)
- Gastrointestinal issues (such as acid reflux)
- Sleep Apnea

Those are only a few of the more common medical conditions that can cause insomnia. Along with those, there can also be neurological conditions (like *Parkinson's Disease or restless leg syndrome)* or a large number of different conflictions that may prevent the brains neurotransmitters from operating correctly.

Aside from medical conditions, many choices that we make, and lifestyle decisions can prevent our brains from being able to calm down and find their sleep state.

- Too much caffeine
- Alcohol (may help to fall asleep, but not stay asleep)
- Graveyard shifts at work
- Working from home
- Diet (not just what you eat, but when)

Then there are the mental reasons for developing insomnia.

- Depression
- Tension
- Anxiety
- Overall worrying (about the past and future)

Every mental reason for people not being able to fall asleep all boil down to one point; not being able to silence the chatter and turn the brain off. Of course, it doesn't really shutdown when going to sleep but that is how you should think of it if a mental reason is the cause for your insomnia. If you are dealing with depression or any other mental condition and believe that it is linked to your insomnia then you should consult the proper professional source along with using the herbs listed in this book. Either way, if you can find a way to silence the mental noise and fall asleep, that will only help to alleviate your insomnia as well. It may be a struggle but know that it can be done. Remember that you are not alone in dealing with this problem. It is the oldest confliction to trouble mankind, and there has always been a collection of natural herbs to help you and everyone overcome these hurdles.

Nature vs Pharmacy

Over-the-counter sleeping aids are one of the most common things people reach for when trying to move out of the pattern of insomnia. Pharmaceutical sleeping aids do have their place, if they didn't work to some extent then people wouldn't spend billions of dollars on them every year. Over-the-counter sleep aids are not all they are cracked up to be though. The list of side effects for anyone of them can be staggering to read through. In the long run, a pharmaceutical sleep aid can actually serve to hurt your sleeping pattern and lock you deeper into a cycle of insomnia. This can happen because sleep aids can be addicting. When someone stops taking the sleep aid, they will notice that they can't fall back asleep, and then start taking the sleep aid again.

All-natural herbs on the other hand, when used correctly, are safe from these problems. Herbs are a substance directly handed down to us from Mother Nature herself. She has placed down these gifts for us so that we can, while navigating the courses of our daily lives, get the proper rest we all need. Much in the same way that many people take sleep for granted, the herbs that have always been with us tend to be neglected as well. Or, and possibly more common, they have not so much been neglected as they have just been unknown. When you know what herbs to use, you won't need to reach for the sleeping pills anymore.

Chapter 2:

Setting the Circadian Clock

Living organisms have a built-in internal clock that we are all born with. It is called the circadian clock. This birth given time piece helps our bodies to distinguish between the external and internal functions of our physiology based around the 24 hours of the day. There was a time, long ago before we were surrounded by light bulbs and electrical devices, where the circadian clocks of most people were left to settle themselves out without any active intervention on anyone's part. Then as technology advanced, we have slowly introduced a steady string of unnatural frequencies into our bodies and threw off the stability and integrity of our circadian clocks. Computer screens, tablets, even the cell phones most of us carry around all day can send subtle and sinuous currents into our bodies and confuse our internal functions to the point where our circadian clocks don't really know what time it is anymore. These items, the computers and cell phones, should not be thought of as anything negative, for they do add helpful conveniences into our daily lives, but they do come with a tradeoff of misaligning our circadian clocks.

Not everything regarding the circadian clock has to do with modern technology though. Everyone is different, and the genes we are born with also have a factor in determining how well our circadian clocks operate. Somewhere up to 15 different genes have an effect in how our circadian clocks function from person to person. Some people are morning people while others will feel more clarity and surges of energy during the nighttime hours. Our individual circadian clocks will tell our bodies when it's time for rest, or, when we should get up and expend our energy.

Even though we are born with different gears inside our internal clocks, many people today don't even realize that theirs has been thrown out of loop with nature. Long hours at work, fighting against sleep to get other things done, jetlag, and a host of other factors can confuse our circadian clocks and thus, lead to insomnia. Even something as simple as having a small bite to eat in the later hours of the evening can confuse our clocks. When the circadian clock begins to get confused, it will still do what it can to regulate itself and possibly make a biological miscalculation while doing so. As with many of the other reasons that can cause insomnia, the vicious loop of not being able to quiet our minds and ease our bodies when we should be asleep can begin without any of us even realizing that a problem has begun.

It can be difficult to figure out if any of this has happened to you and determine for a fact that having a confused circadian clock is contributing to your lack of sleep at night. Just so you know, if you live in our modern age (which you obviously do) and have trouble sleeping at night, then your circadian clock is properly at least somewhat maladjusted. This is nothing to feel down about as it is just a spandrel of the age and times we live in. Almost everyone has a maladjusted circadian clock nowadays. Yet, again, our biological time piece doesn't realize that something is wrong. It's not up to the circadian clock to be completely accurate and fix itself, for that will keep on ticking and tracking time along with our organs as it sees fit. It is up to us to reset the circadian clock, after recognizing that is has been thrown out of synch with the sun and moon.

Even if you don't have an inaccurate circadian clock, you should go about making sure that it ticks along as correctly as possible. To do this, you will have to reset your circadian clock and get it back on the proper time track with Mother Nature. Quick fix fads that guarantee to solve everything for you probably won't do what they claim, except take your money. Also, any pill for the most part will not correctly set your circadian clock to its proper state either. In fact, depending on what the pill is, like a sleeping pill, they will only cause to confuse your biological time tracker even more. The exceptions to this are melatonin and magnesium- which are both natural supplements and are produced inside our bodies.

Both melatonin and magnesium can help to ease muscles and relax the mind. Melatonin is often recommended when trying to induce more sleep by the medical community. Using either one of these correctly can help to reset your circadian clock, but there are other tips that you can start practicing even before reaching for those supplements.

How to reset the circadian clock

The most fundamental way to get back in tune with nature is to be aligned with the sun and moon. This is practical and conventional wisdom. We receive all of our energy from the sun and its light. Moonlight, valuable in its own regard, is only a reflection and does not send down surges of energy into our molecular cells. We should live the course of our lives with the basic system of sunlight and moonlight engrained into our minds at all times. When it is daytime, things should be bright, and during the night, things should be dark. Both, light and darkness, are necessary for our bodies to function properly.

When waking up in the morning (or just getting out of bed if you couldn't get any sleep) the first thing you should do is surround yourself with as much light as possible. Open the blinds and let the light flood your room. Open the window while you are at it to bring in some fresh air (remember that the sun also help supply oxygen). If you can, take a step outside before getting most other things done and just take a brief moment to wrap yourself in sunlight, and feel appreciation for it. Turn the lights on all over your house, especially in the room you woke up in. If you wake up very early before the sun has fully rose, it's raining outside, or the clouds are covering the sunlight, then you are going to have to rely on artificial light even more to help get your circadian clock back in proper tune with nature. Artificial light may not be as energy inducing, and of course not as natural, as sunlight, but it is better than wallowing the morning hours away while covered in darkness. The brighter your surroundings are after waking up, the more you are telling your body and mind that it is time to use energy and become lucid. If after first getting up and everything is dark, then you are sending the exact opposite message to your circadian clock. This can be one of the major reasons why many people don't feel refreshed and ready to go after getting out of bed. They wake up, and both their bodies and minds still think that it's time to get rest and slow down instead of taking action and speed up.

This same logic applies to nighttime as well. During the night it is better to lower the lights and lessen the energy. Our society is counterintuitive to this concept, in some locations. Cities are primarily guilty of creating environments where the cycle of day and night is mixed-up. Living within a *"City that never sleeps"* is not the best place to be when trying to combat insomnia. Of course, living in a city does not mean there is no hope, but if you do then it may take a little bit longer to reset your circadian clock back to being in tune with Mother Nature. If you do live in a city or some other highly populated area with a vibrant and active nightlife, be aware that you may have to put in a bit of extra effort and have patience. Remember that sleep is to be taken seriously and some of your nighttime adventures may need to be put on pause while you are trying to reset your circadian clock.

When night comes it is best to lower the volume of light surrounding you. You don't need to drape your home in total darkness but dimming the lights will begin to tell your body that it does not need to expend as much energy. Have less lights on and if you can then only try to use a few lamps. If your lights have dim switches and lower settings, use those after the sun goes down.

During the day, have your home and environment emulate the sun. During the night, emulate the moon.

By doing this you will be on the way to having your body and mind emulate our most intrinsic celestial bodies, then you will be on your way to getting your circadian clock back in the proper tune with Mother Nature.

What to Do at Night

As it gets closer to bedtime you can perform a variety of different things to wind yourself down and inform the circadian clock that the time to go to sleep is getting closer. One of the best ways to accomplish this is to take a warm bath an hour or so before trying to get some sleep. Taking a warm bath has a tendency to calm the mind and relax the body. Also, warming up the body will begin to let muscles ease tension and relax.

Turn off all electric lights when it is time to go to sleep. Computers, cell phones, televisions, tablets, video game systems, and whatever else that may produce blue or red lights should be shutdown. You may even want to take the extra step and unplug these things to stifle any electric currents that may be disrupting your sleep without you even realizing it.

Don't worry, when morning comes you can turn everything back on and use all the devices you want to your hearts content.

Read a book in bed or write in a journal before going to sleep. Doing these things *in bed* is key here. Reading can help to focus the mind and slow it down while at the same time putting it to a little bit extra work of processing information. Journaling can help to organize the activities and thoughts of the day that may be preventing you from quieting the mind while trying to fall asleep. If you read or write using an electrical device, just be sure to turn it off after you have finished.

Both reading, and writing can also give you something to focus on while you transition from being awake into subconsciousness, and that leads to another tip. When trying to sleep, it is not advisable to have your thoughts scattered all over the place, as that will only keep the mind too active. When trying to sleep, either focus on a memory (like a conversation) or play out a sequence in your head. The sequence could also be a memory, or even something you saw in a movie. It's also not the worst idea to let your imagination run away a tad while trying to go to sleep. Whatever your wildest fantasies may be, go ahead and envision yourself accomplishing them.

Regular exercise can do wonders for fixing the circadian clock. Try to exercise at least 45 minutes, four days out of the week. But, don't exercise right before going to sleep as that will rev you up too much.

Meditation is an excellent thing to do before going to bed. It can help to calm the mind and center your thoughts before bed.
Try not to have any caffeine 6 hours before bedtime. Also, watch the carbs after 9 pm.

Get a routine before going to bed. Having a set routine will, after a week or two, let your circadian clock know that it is time to wind down and get some shuteye.

Chapter 3:

Sleeping with Plants

It is no secret that being close to nature can help to settle down the nerves and bring a calming energy to the mind. When trying to tune in closer to Mother Nature's frequency the best thing you can do without question is spend time outside in the sunlight and take in as much of her splendor as you can. Going on a hiking trail, a park, or simply just gardening in your own yard all have the ability to bring a Zenlike breath of air into just about anybody's day. Not all of us have access to such things though and may have to travel very far if we decided to get more in touch with the beauty of our natural world.

If you can't easily sperate yourself from the rat race and frantic trappings of an unnatural environment, if you can't easily go and get back in touch with Mother Nature, you can still bring her a little closer to you! Trust me when I tell you that she won't mind, and also trust that just by adding a few plants to your domicile can help to lower stress and even make your home healthier.

A less illustrated and chronicled reason for insomnia sneaking up on us may be related to the quality of our indoor air. If you can't properly breath during the night then getting to sleep will only be that much harder. Even if you are a devout neat freak an assortment of different molds and odors can start to grow within our homes and go unrecognized for far too long. These things can lower the quality of our air the same way that normal air pollution can. That's another one to watch out for, air pollution. It is probably seeping in from the outside and into your bedroom without you ever being the wiser to it. Yet research studies have shown, even a particular one performed by NASA, that plants can help to purify the air that we breath. Just simply being around plants, and taking the time to properly care for them, can induce a sense of wellbeing along with clearing out our airwaves. When it comes to reducing mental stress, one of the answers is literally all around us in the world of plants.

If you think that your trouble with sleeping at night is more mental than physical then you may want to start investing in some plant life and placing them all over your home. Specifically, place plants in the room that you normally sleep in. Going the extra mile would be to grow the plants from scratch inside your bedroom, but that may not be applicable for everyone, and understandably so. Even if it is not, don't fret. There are a large number of different plants that you can find and set down in your bedroom without having to grow them from scratch. Just remember to treat the plants with kindness and take care of them correctly, do not neglect them. After all, aside from being a part of Mother Nature, they are helping to calm your nerves and clear the air of toxins- both of which will help you sleep better at night.

Golden Pothos

This plant has also been called "Devil's Ivy" but don't let that trick you into avoiding it. This plant does have leaves that are slightly toxic, but it is also a very good plant to hang so it stays out of reach of children or animals. It is easy to care for however and is very handy at clearing out the air of pollutants. They can grow up to roughly around 30 feet indoors, so some pruning may be required. Within containers it shouldn't grow more than 10 feet. It has a vine, ivy, like appearance and is not susceptible to many pests, but every now and then may become infested with some bugs. It should be noted that the leaves should not ever be ingested.

Jasmine

This fan favorite has been shown to lower anxiety and promote better sleep. Using Jasmine plants to sleep better is nothing new and has been practiced for thousands of years. They also have glorious ivory or pink blossoms and are certainly easy on the eyes. They won't bloom at all if they don't receive enough cool temperature though, so keep that in mind. They also can, sometimes, grow rather wildly so pruning should be done regularly. Seeing as these plants can be enthusiastic climbers, an indoor trellis is recommended for them. They also are known to live for a long time when properly taken care of. They can be susceptible to infestation from mealybugs, keep an eye out for that.

Gerbera Daisies

It can be a bit difficult to not feel your spirits brighten when looking at this bright white, pink, yellow, and orange flower. They can also directly help to combat insomnia since during the night they release oxygen which will help to breathe easier. A word of warning is needed for these plants though; they are not the easiest to care for and not recommended to novices. They do require sunlight, but not direct or too much of it. Seeing as how beautiful they are, it can be hard to not want to place them in your homes, but before selecting this plant do some extra research and make sure you can properly give it everything it needs.

Lavender

Many would consider this one to be the champion of the plant world when it comes to defeating insomnia. It has the double-edged power of both reducing anxiety and inducing sleep. It has been proven to slow the heart rate down and lower blood pressure as well. The scent of Lavender is world renowned, and for good reason. Simply smelling the delicate aroma may be all it takes to relax and ease into a better state for finding sleep.

Lavender is a moderate plant to care for. It may require pruning once a year and needs to be watered in different cycles relating to its age, but the benefits from making this plant one of your roommates can't be emphasized enough.

Snake Plant

Also known as "Mother-in-law's Tongue". That may be an odd nickname for a plant to have but don't be distracted by it. This is a great plant for beginners as it does not take much botanical knowledge to take proper care of it. They are also known to be hardy plants, so novices can be assured that even though they may be new to the world of living with plants, the Snake Plant will be able to endure whatever rookie mistakes they might make.

This should be one of your go to choices when choosing a plant to help alleviate insomnia. First, know that this plant emits oxygen during the evening hours which will start to clear the airways of where ever you slumber. Second, it also soaks up the carbon dioxide that is floating around us (carbon dioxide is something that we emit while breathing). Third, the

Snake Plant has been proven to remove some of the common but unwanted toxins that are already floating through most homes such as; benzene, trichloroethylene, and formaldehyde. If all of that weren't enough, just know that a Snake Plant can be purchased already potted and ready to go. Sizes may slightly vary but acquiring a typical 6-inch potted Snake Plant should not be hard to find. All you have to do is find it, buy it, and set it. It is already to go right out of the gate.

Valerian

Pink, white, and the sweet scent of summer are just some of the ways to describe this plant. Even better, this plant has an ancient history when it comes to staving off insomnia. Galen, the famed Roman philosopher and physician, specifically used to prescribe Valerian root to rid his patients of insomnia. The modern research of today has caught up to Galen and promotes his claims from so long ago. According to some people, just inhaling the scent of Valerian root is enough to bring on a comfortable night of sound sleep. The herb of Valerian root will come in very handy when combating insomnia, but simply having a flower of it in your room can also kick your fight against insomnia into the next level. In the long-lost days were practicing magic was a common occurrence Valerian was used to construct dream pillows- just another cultural association between Valerian and getting some good sleep.

We could go all day about the different cultural and scientific links between Valerian and getting solid sleep, but it would take a whole entire other book to do so. It hasn't been labeled a medical wonder plant for no reason. All you should know before adding it to your living space is that it is a moderate plant to care for, so extra research may be required, and it is not recommended for people who spend a lot of time around horses, as it is not best for them.

Aloe Vera

This is another plant with a longstanding history in ancient cultures (it was dubbed by the Egyptians as a plant of immortality). The plant has a cactus like appearance, but it is also one of the easiest plants to care for and is fine for novices. Although neglecting plants is not recommended, if your busy life causes you to forget to take care of your plant now and then, Aloe Vera will be able to handle itself just fine. It has a strong will to live and reproduces itself quite easily, so if you only start out with one then you will soon have enough to place in every room of the house, and maybe even be able to give away a few as surprise gifts.

NASA thinks very highly of Aloe Vera as well. They even went so far as to dub it one of the best plants to improve overall air quality. During the evening Aloe Vera releases oxygen into the air which will undoubtedly help you to get a better night's rest. If you are unsure which plant to get to help you sleep, don't want to take up too much space, or are lacking a green thumb, then this is certainly the one you should first add to your home and bedroom.

Precautions of living with plants

Although having plants in your home and bedroom can be very beneficial to reducing insomnia, there are a few precautions to keep in mind. If you have pets or children then make sure that the plants are not toxic to them. Knowing what is dangerous to certain animals, and your children's medical history, should always be first priority. It should also be mentioned that different people have different taste, so it is not just important to acquire plants whose appearance you appreciate, but also consider the aromas they give off and be sure that they are pleasurable to your sense of smell. You also will have to keep up with taking proper care of the plants, which involves a little bit more then watering them and making sure they get the proper sunlight. Be mindful to, at least once a week, clean the leaves by carefully wiping them. Making sure the leaves are clean will not just make the plants healthier but will also help them to do their job of keeping the air in your home purified. You help them, and they will help you, as goes the reciprocal balance of Mother Nature and all her precious children.

There are a number of different plants that can help to clean the air and bring on a better night's sleep but the once listed above are some of the best that you will be able to find without having to have a deep understanding of taking care of plants. Invite Mother Nature into your home and sleep easier after doing it.

Chapter 4:

The 10 Best Herbs for Sleeping Better

The world is overflowing with natural herbs. There are thousands, if not more, medicinal herbs in the natural world and these are the 10 best ones for getting better sleep.

Herbs, like modern medicine, do come with some warnings. If you are concerned with how these herbs may affect you, consult with your health care provider before taking any of these herbs.

These herbs are not appearing in any order of performance or superiority as not one of them is thoroughly better than any other. Use them one at a time or in conjunction with each other. Experiment and find out which ones you like best and help you the most.

Ashwagandha (Withania somnifera)

This herb is a part of the nightshade family. It originates from the dry regions of Yemen, China, and Nepal. It is a part of the species, *somnifera*, which can be translated to "sleep inducing" in Latin. The root powder of the plant has been used in traditional Indian medicine for centuries to combat several maladies, including insomnia. Modern scientific studies, including one done at the Sleep Institute in Japan, have confirmed that Ashwagandha does in fact bring about sleep, but exactly how and why remains unknown. Although exactly why Ashwagandha brings about peaceful sleep in unknown, it may have something to do with the water extract of the leaf being rich in triethylene glycol (TEG) which has been shown to reduce non-rapid eye movement (NREM). It has also been shown to reduce cortisol levels.

Ashwagandha should not be used by pregnant women. It may also aggravate symptoms of the following; thyroid disorders, lupus, multiple sclerosis, stomach ulcers, unbalanced blood pressure.

This herb is commonly consumed by brewing it in a tea. The standard dosage is 6000 milligrams a day (taken 3 times a day) or 100 milligrams when used in a cup of tea. It can also be purchased in supplement form.

Its appearance is orange or red, and a plum like bud.

California Poppy (Eschscholzia californica)

California Poppy is a resident of both Mexico and California. Also known as the "Cup of gold", this famed herb has even become the official state flower of California.

The side effects for using this herb to get over insomnia are minimal. It is still being researched how this herb may affect women during pregnancy, so it is better to avoid using it while pregnant. It also may slow down the nervous system too much, which is fine for sleeping but is not recommended for use if you have any sort of surgery coming up as it may conflict with anesthetics. Stop using this herb two weeks prior to any surgery. It should also be noted that the dosages for this herb can vary depending on age and other factors, so follow directions that come along with the herb carefully.

California Poppy has been shown to reduce a large collection of different nighttime aches while also slowing down the nervous system. These two factors combined can easily lead someone into falling asleep. Major ingredients within this herb are isoquinoline alkaloids. These alkaloids bind to serotonin and opioid receptors (this herb is not an opiate). Stimulating the opioid receptors is what blocks the pain and activating the serotonin receptors is what brings on the sleep.

It is commonly used in tea or can be purchased as an extract.

This herb has a very bright and sunny appearance, coming in different shades of yellow, orange, red, and on a rare occasion even pink.

Cordyceps (Cordyceps sinensis)

Cordyceps name is a combination of the Greek word for "club" and the Latin word for "head". Cordyceps are a fungus that grows all over Asia and have been used for medicinal purposes for ages.

Pregnant women should not eat Cordyceps. They can also, on rare occasions, cause diarrhea or upset the stomach but only when taken in large doses.

Cordyceps have been proven to dilatate the airways for our lungs, which allows more oxygen to reach our blood and induce sleep. Besides that, they also have shown to give boosts of energy and help athletes when training. Getting better sleep is only one of the benefits of eating Cordyceps. When taking them before bed they will induce a sedative like action and help to receive a deeper sleep. Seeing as this mushroom comes with a huge host of health benefits you should start adding it into your diet.

Cordyceps mushrooms are not known for tasting very good. When ingested they are usually powdered and dried out first. You can find them sold in jars and filled with powder, so they can be mixed with water, or you can buy them in the form of tablets.

German Chamomile (Matricaria chamomilla)

This one is well known and quite famous for helping people get better sleep. It has been used for centuries and found much popularity among the Greeks, Romans, and Egyptians. Its popularity hasn't dwindled either as this is still one of the most common herbs people reach for when trying to calm down and fall asleep.

A German study that tested Chamomile on animals showed that it acts as a mild sedative which helps to bring about sleep. A separate study researching Chamomiles affect against anxiety unveiled results that it reduces the symptoms of anxiety for people who have *generalized anxiety disorder* (GED). The gist is, lower doses of Chamomile reduce anxiety while higher doses induce sleep.

Do not ingest Chamomile if you are allergic to ragweed. Pregnant woman should avoid using Chamomile. It is also not recommended to be used in conjunction with NSAIDs (aspirin and other anti-inflammatory drugs).

Chamomile is typically used in a tea. There are a variety of different types of Chamomile that can be purchased and the two that you want to look for are Roman and German. We recommend using the German due to having our own better personal experiences, but that is subjective. Feel free to try both of them. It can also be purchased in capsule form, ointments, or the petals can be placed in bathwater.

Hops (Humulus lupulus)

These flowers are most famous for being used in beer and also being related to cannabis. It is not recommended to drink alcohol to reduce insomnia. You may fall sleep faster, but you may also wake up in the middle of the night. Although smoking cannabis may help bring about sleep, due to the illegality and controversy surrounding it, it is not recommended either.

Hops contain an active ingredient known as 2-methyl-3-buten-2-ol (MB). MB can interact with what is known as the GABA pathway. MB can bind with receptors in the brain and by doing so it can improve the binding of GABA. GABA is very important for falling and staying asleep. People who suffer from insomnia have lower Gaba levels than those who don't. Hops also bind with our melatonin receptors. Melatonin is produced within our brains and is needed for falling asleep. It specifically produces itself when our eyes notice darkness and induces a sleepy feeling. By using Hops, you are binding to your GABA pathway and melatonin, getting a double whammy of neurological chemicals to help you fall asleep.

Pregnant women should avoid ingesting Hops. It should also not be used if you are currently suffering from depression. It may conflict with anesthetics. Stop using this herb two weeks prior to any surgery. It also contains some chemicals that mimic estrogen and as such should not be used for people who are dealing with hormone sensitive cancers or conditions.

An ancient practice using Hops for sleep was to make a pillow out of them. They are also brewed into tea, and in some cases even soft drinks.

Lavender (Lavandula officinalis)

Lavender is a native of the old world and grew almost on a global scale. Its gentle aroma is probably its most famous feature (next to its gorgeous violet appearance).

Several studies across the world have been done on Lavender in conjunction with sleep, although most of the studies were only small in scale. One study done in Thailand showed that Lavender may go so far as altering brain function to something calmer and more peaceful. It also showed a reduction in heart rate, respiratory rate, and blood pressure. Another research done in Britain specially relating to insomnia had several participants sleep in rooms where Lavender essential oil was pumped into the room while they slept at night while another group of people slept in rooms that did not have any Lavender. After a week of doing this the volunteers were polled on which rooms they received better sleep within, and 20 percent of them all agreed that the room with Lavender was superior.

Lavender is usually considered perfectly safe when

ingested via the mouth. It should not be used by women who are pregnant or breastfeeding though. It is also not to be used by young boys who have yet to reach puberty, and it may conflict with anesthetics, so stop using this herb two weeks prior to any surgery.

There are a variety of different ways to use Lavender but it all comes down to the scent and oils. You can place a few drops of oil in a bath, place some of the flowers in a bowl next to your bed, put a few drops on your wrists or neck, spray it into the air before going to bed, or even sprinkle a tad of it on a tissue and place it underneath your pillow. Since Lavender is all about the scent, don't be scared to get a little bit creative with how you decide to use it.

Lemon Balm (Melissa officinalis)

Lemon Balm is a member of the mint family. It originates from parts of Asia, south-central Europe, the Mediterranean, and Iran. It has been used both to reduce pain and as a sleep aid ever since the Dark Ages

Lemon Balm contains something called eugenol. If

you have ever been to a dentist then you have had this before, as it is what they use to numb a patient before doing work on the mouth. Eugenol is not just a numbing agent but can also help induce sleep. It is used to combat insomnia, and for people who don't have insomnia it is used to sleep longer. It has also been shown to reduce the symptoms of both anxiety and overall stress.

Lemon Balm should not be used by woman who are pregnant or breastfeeding. It also should not be used by people who have the following conditions; thyroid disease, diabetes, or anyone who has a surgery scheduled within two weeks. Infants should not use Lemon Balm for more than four weeks. When taken by the mouth it may cause the following; dizziness, stomach pain, nausea, increased appetite. When applied to the skin it may act as an irritant.

Lemon Balm can be brewed in a tea (hot and iced are both used for Lemon Balm) but is also normally combined with Valerian root. While this herb can be used on its own, it is normally combined with other herbs and a variety of foods (it is a common and popular ice-cream topping). Candies, fruits, and even fish (have you ever eaten Lemon Balm pesto?) have been combined with Lemon Balm. A little extra tip when wanting to use Lemon Balm, mix it in a spearmint tea.

It can also be used for aromatherapy, as an oil, or applied externally.

Passionflower (Passiflora)

Passionflower can be found growing in Oceania, the United States, Southeast Asia, the Central and South Americas, and Mexico. This flower and vine is most known for producing the popular *Passion Fruit*. It also turns out that Passionflower has been used to treat several different health issues for many a number of years and between the 18th and 20th century it shot up in popularity and usage. Before that it was used by the Houma, Aztecs, and Cherokee people for fighting anxiety and getting better sleep.

It also has a rich, hidden, history. Legend says that while Spanish explores were adventuring through the Peruvian landscape they saw the Christian cross (Passion of the cross) hidden within the flower on multiple occasions.

Different studies have shown that by drinking Passionflower tea for 7 days may help to reduce anxiety as well as bring on a better night's sleep. This is another herb that can boost GABA levels in the brain, which is needed when trying to combat against insomnia. It has also been shown to relax nerves.

A study conducted in 2011 tested 41 participants by using Passionflower as compared to other items that can cause a placebo effect. Insomnia was one of the conditions that was specifically looked into. The results; those who used Passionflower claimed to have better results overcoming insomnia as compared to the other placebos.

In 2013 another study was done comparing three of the herbs in this list (Hops, Valerian, and Passionflower) against common pharmaceutical sleep aides. It was concluded that at the end of trial that the herbs did just as well, if not better, then the pharmaceutical drugs. Yet, none of the herbs showed to have addictive properties.

Stop using this herb two weeks prior to any surgery as it may conflict with anesthesia. Pregnant women should not use Passionflower. The effects of Passionflower while breastfeeding is inconclusive and thus should not be used. Also, when taken in large amounts, Passionflower may cause the following when taken via the mouth in large doses; nausea, inflamed blood vessels, an altered state of consciousness, confusion, dizziness, and irregular muscles action and coordination.

Passionflower is commonly brewed in teas. Most health food stores sell dried Passionflower and even already made, prepackaged, tea mixes. It can also be bought in capsules, tablets, and liquid extracts.

Siberian Ginseng (Eleutherococcus senticosus)

Everyone has heard of ginseng. The Chinese have been aggressively promoting the mountain sized list of benefits that ginseng offers to the human race for eons. The Russian people also have their own form of ginseng, and for ages it has been used to help people fall asleep. Just because it is also called "Devils shrub" should not scare you off from giving it an honest try. Also, be aware that Siberian Ginseng is not a true ginseng, as it does not contain ginsenosides. Don't let that stop you either, as this herb has been labeled as a superfood.

Unfortunately, not many research studies have been done on Siberian Ginseng and its fame for reducing insomnia has spread more from word of mouth. That word of mouth has spread far though and in many circles this is one of the main herbs used to getting better sleep. It has also been extolled to fight off fatigue, boost energy, increase sexual functions, and is an anti-inflammatory.

Siberian Ginseng should not be used by women who are breastfeeding or pregnant. It also should not be used by anyone who has the following conditions; Diabetes, schizophrenia or mania, high blood pressure, heart conditions, cancer, or any bleeding disorder.

There are a huge number of different ways that you can take and use Siberian Ginseng. As with most herbs, it can be brewed in a tea on its own or combined with other herbs. You can also find it available as an extract, a supplement, a powder, or you can even find fresh Siberian Ginseng at a large variety of health food stores. If you have trouble locating it then check out some Asian food markets or order some online.

Valerian (Valeriana officinalis)

This lovely pink plant is a native to both Asia and Europe. Both the Romans and Greeks used Valerian often to combat against lack of sleep and lowering anxiety.

The National Institutes of Health have claimed that Valerian has a several different chemical compounds that work together to produce sedative properties. A separate group, the European Medicines Agency (EMA), approved of a health claim that Valerian can both produce sleep and act to reduce mild nervous tension when used as a dried extract.

Although exactly why Valerian works for battling insomnia is currently lacking clarity, it is most likely another herb that helps to increase GABA in the brain. It is believed that Valerian promotes GABA growth in two different ways. It may block an enzyme that destroys GABA, and by doing so more GABA can come in to help you fall asleep. The other thing that it is believed to do is release more GABA into your system. Not only is it producing more GABA, but it is blocking the forces that try to remove GABA. The hard science is still looking into this, but is it any wonder why Valerian has been used for besting the demon of insomnia for so long? In fact, even though many from the scientific community are still looking into the effects of Valerian, it is a common recommendation for weening people off of sleeping pills and falling back in tune with Mother Nature.

There is a window of time that should be taken into consideration when using Valerian though. 2-3 weeks are the magic numbers. Try using Valerian for only 2-3 weeks, then take a break for another 2-3 weeks before starting to use it again.

Valerian should not be used by women who are breastfeeding or are pregnant. Its usage should also be stopped two weeks prior to any surgery. It is also not advisable to give to children who are 3 years old or younger. The rest of the side effects are minimal. It may cause any of the following; excitability, heart disturbances, mental dullness, dizziness, uneasiness, upset stomach, or headaches.

The part of the herb that is used to reduce insomnia is the root. Thankfully, there are several different ways to harness the power of Valerian without having to dig it up. As with most herbs it can be brewed in a tea. It can also be bought in the forms of capsules, tinctures, or tablets.

Chapter 5:

Herbal Teas

When dealing with natural herbs, the question of how to properly ingest them may arise. Different cultures that have relied on herbs for medicinal use, to overcome insomnia and other problems, have their own methods, opinions, and traditions. In some situations, the herbs have been either eaten or smoked. When dealing with insomnia and aiming to use herbs to fall asleep though, brewing them into a tea is a tried and true tradition that has not only withstood the test of time but is still being added onto in our current day and age. Modern research is constantly backing up what some of the ancient masters always knew and recommended; use tea to get better sleep.

Before turning in to go to sleep is the best time to drink a cup of tea when using it to defeat insomnia. Different sources will give different directions for how to brew and drink it. It should go without saying, but the best way to brew your own tea is with a teapot, not some newfangled electronic device that will do all the work for you. It will be far easier for you to learn what works for you by doing it yourself. The thing to remember about tea is, it all comes down to the taste. You are free to alter these recipes and find out what works and tastes best to you.

There are two recommended ways to drink these teas after you brewed them. The first is to drink a full medium cup a half an hour before going to bed. The second is to drink several small amounts at your leisure several hours before bed. Experiment and see which method you enjoy more.

Unless otherwise stated, brew the teas listed here for 20 minutes after placing all the ingredients in. All water should be boiled beforehand. You can try to ice some of these teas if you want, but when doing so it will weaken the therapeutic effects and remember that a warmer body is more likely to fall asleep. Also, they really don't taste the same when iced.

All herbs should be strained before adding them to the tea.

There are a few light warnings to go over before diving into the different tea blends.

- Tea is not for young child. This is more or less a choice left up to the parents, but to be on the safe side, children should avoid partaking in stimulants.
- Tea should not be consumed by women who are currently pregnant.
- It is not safe to combine some teas and herbs with certain medications. If you are unsure, don't risk drinking any tea. Consult your doctor before doing anything else.

Easy Going Sleepy Time Tea Blend

This is sometimes known as "Simple Blend". It is an easy mixture that just about anyone will be able to brew even without having much experience making their own tea. As this is the first recipe there are not many details, you can add or take away what sort of herbs you want in it.

- 2 tablespoons of any sort of tea blend (non-caffeinated)

- 1 cup of boiling water
- Any amount and combination of strained herbs. The most common method is to use an equal amount of lavender and chamomile. Try one tablespoon of each and see how it works for you. If the taste doesn't agree with you, or if you don't receive the affects you want, try adding some different herbs, reduce the amount of either the lavender or chamomile, or increase one over the either.

Relaxing Tea Blend

This tea has a very interesting ingredient in it that I'm sure you will notice quickly.

- 1 cup of boiling water
- 1 teaspoon of catnip (yes people put this in tea, and have been doing so since the 1700's)
- 1 tablespoon of Valerian
- 1 tablespoon of Hops
- 1 tablespoon of Lemon Balm
- 2 tablespoons of Chamomile

Rest Easy Tea Blend

This tea is loaded with an assortment of different herbs to calm you down and rest easy.

- 1 cup of boiling water
- 1 and a half tablespoons of Hops
- 1 tablespoon of Passionflower
- 1 tablespoon of Oats
- 3 tablespoons of Chamomile

Miracle Tea Blend

This tea is a super sleep inducer. It will probably knock you out, but it has a heavy taste. Don't say you weren't warned.

- 1 cup of boiling water
- 1 tablespoon of Valerian
- 1 tablespoon of Lavender
- 2 tablespoons of Hops
- 3 tablespoons of Passionflower
- 3 tablespoons of Lemon Balm

Banana Cinnamon Tea

This tea is not a so-called herbal tea, but it is still all natural and will help calm you down to get the proper sleep you need. Ingesting some cinnamon can help even out blood sugar levels. Blood sugar, when too high or low, can disrupt part of your biological process and keep you awake longer then you want, or wake you up in the middle of the night. Another thing that you may not be aware of is that the peel part of the banana is actually loaded with magnesium and potassium. The peel actually has more magnesium then the part of the banana that we usually eat. Both magnesium and potassium can help ease the muscles, which will help you get better sleep. This recipe also contains Stevia. Stevia will help to sweeten the drink and will also help balance out your blood sugar, and it won't spike your blood sugar before going to sleep. To top it all off, it is a unique tea, and is very easy to brew.

- 1 cup of boiling water
- 1 banana, with the peel. Cut both ends of the banana in half (the top and bottom) and toss them in with the water. Slice the peel up into

several tiny pieces and toss them in as well.

- A pinch of cinnamon
- You should only boil this tea for ten minutes
- Add a pinch of Stevia
- Pour a cup and add more cinnamon if you desire

Chapter 6:

Naturally Beating Insomnia

When dealing with insomnia, taking in too much information at once can often seem staggering. For that reason, a comprehensive list of the top 10 best tips for beating your insomnia and getting back in tune with Mother Nature has been compiled for you. If ever confused, or just need a refresher, then simply just come back to this chapter and find out everything you need to know. Best of luck to you overcoming insomnia and reestablishing your relationship with Mother Nature.

Number 1: Use the herbs

Use the herbs in this book located in chapter 4. Learn more about them on your own and experiment to see which ones work best for you. Here are the best herbs used to beat insomnia;

- **Ashwagandha**
- **California Poppy**
- **Cordyceps**
- **German Chamomile**
- **Hops**
- **Lavender**
- **Lemon Balm**
- **Passionflower**
- **Siberian Ginseng**
- **Valerian**

Number 2: Drink Tea

Drink a cup of tea a day, preferably before going to bed.

Number 3: Take Sleep Seriously

Understand why you have fallen into the pattern of insomnia in the first place.

Number 4: Exercise and Meditate

Both of these activities will help to center both the

body and mind. They will also go a very long way in getting your circadian clock back on its proper track. Exercise will increase blood flow and, when laying down to sleep, you will feel a quicker sensation of sleep taking you over. By exercising during the day, your body will better understand exactly what muscles to restore and functions to focus on while you sleep.

Meditation is the most natural method of clearing up any mental issue, including insomnia. Not only will practicing the different breathing exercises help to control your heart rate and increase oxygen, meditating (even for 5 minutes a day) will also help to clear your thoughts and organize all the action going on in your mind that you were never even aware about. Although exercise and meditation can give you a healthy boost on their own, using them in conjunction with each other is a formula that can't be beaten. Just remember not to exercise too late at night, as that may keep you up longer.

Number 5: Melatonin and Magnesium

Most people don't realize that these two vital components that are needed for sleep are lacking in their bodies. Magnesium deficiency and a lack of melatonin being produced in the brain are more common than most people think. Check with your doctor to see if you are lacking either one of these, and then get a supplement to bring everything back in proper order.

Number 6: Sleep with Plants

Hang some plants in your home, especially the room that you go to sleep in. Doing so will not just clear the air, purify toxins, but will also replicate the great outdoors and you will be welcoming Mother Nature into your home with you. She is a fantastic roommate to bunk with.

Here is the list of plants to store in your home for quick reference;

- **Golden Pothos**
- **Jasmine**

- **Gerbera Daisies**
- **Lavender**
- **Snake Plant**
- **Valerian**
- **Aloe Vera**

Number 7: Read or Write in Bed

Writing and reading are the best activities to do before sleeping. Both of them will help to focus your mind while not placing it into a state of too much rapid thought. When doing either of these in bed, you are sending a direct message to your body that it is just about time to go to sleep.

Number 8: Get A Routine Before Bed

Creating a ritual and sticking to it, for about two weeks, will eventually cue your body that the time for sleep is approaching. You will notice that the longer you stick to the routine, you will start getting more tired before your routine has even finished. Taking a warm bath, then reading or writing in bed, are some great ways to get your nighttime routine started.

Number 9: Bright Days and Dark Nights

Emulate the sun and moon. During the day, surround yourself with light and try to remain active. During the night, lower the lights and slow down the energy. Also remember to kill off all electric lights (especially the blue ones) before going to bed. Keep in mind that your circadian clock will not reset itself all on its own. You have to be aligned with the sun and moon for it to return to its proper rhythm.

Number 10: Stop Reaching for The Pills

They may work in the short-term but when taken for too long they will only cause to increase your insomnia if you become addicted to them. Drop the pills. They are not one of the many gifts Mother Nature has bestowed upon us. Grab the plants and herbs, as that is what she has grown naturally on our planet Earth. To get back in touch with Mother Nature, use the resources she wants you to.

A final note

Now that you have gone through the entire book and reached the end you can stop and take a breather.

Mother Nature will be very pleased that you have put in so much effort to learn more about her abundant bounty of heavenly and natural gifts. She has and will always be on your side. Yet, she is very busy trying to keep the planet (and the whole entire universe along with the spacetime continuum) alive at all times and, as much as you may not want to hear it, it is up to every single one of us as individuals to make the effort to stay on her good side. It is not up to her to come knocking on our door. No, it is the other way around. As it was already said, she will always be there for each and every single one of us, but we have to go to her.

Our modern day societies do not make this an easy task to complete. If anything, it seems like the runaround ways that society operates wants to keep us away from Mother Nature. This does not seem like it will change anytime soon either. So, as you partake in the herbs and get some well deserved better sleep, remember to keep up your effort to become closer to Mother Nature. By doing so, you will get a whole slew of other benefits then just better sleep out of it.

Conclusion

Thank for making it through to the end of *Herbal Medicine Insomnia: The 10 Best Solutions to Solve Insomnia Naturally*, let's hope it was informative and able to provide you with all of the tools you need to achieve your goals whatever they may be.

The next step is to get ready to do some shopping. Head on out to your local stores, or search online, and get your herbs ready to lead you into a world of sound sleep that you never knew of before! While you are out there grabbing your Lavender, Passionflower, Hops, and all the rest, be sure to pick up a few plants to hang in your home and bedroom along the way. Don't forget about making sure you have a teapot ready to go either or else when trying to brew some delicious and sleep-inducing tea, you'll be out of luck.

Start getting yourself, and your circadian clock, back in proper tune with Mother Nature and then you will wonder why you ever had problems sleeping in the first place. Just always remember that insomnia can sneak up on you again if you do not remain vigilant to keep it away. The herbs and tips in this book are not simply onetime quick fixes but long-lasting solutions that will continue to work as long as you continue to uphold them.

Rest easy and have sweet dreams.

Finally, if you found this book useful in any way, a review on Amazon is always appreciated!

This book belongs to a series of books about herbal medicine and how to use it to improve our life. For more information, visit www.db-publishing.com

www.ingramcontent.com/pod-product-compliance
Lightning Source LLC
Chambersburg PA
CBHW070112260726
48658CB00001B/89